Stay Well
Every Year
of Your Life:

Dr. Molner's
Guide to Total Health

Stay Well
Every Year
of Your Life:

Dr. Molner's
Guide to Total Health

by Joseph Molner, M.D.

PRENTICE-HALL, INC., *Englewood Cliffs, N.J.*

© 1964 by Prentice-Hall, Inc.
Englewood Cliffs, N.J.

Copyright under International and Pan-American Copyright Conventions

T 84634

PRENTICE-HALL INTERNATIONAL, INC., *London*
PRENTICE-HALL OF AUSTRALIA, PTY., LTD., *Sydney*
PRENTICE-HALL OF CANADA, LTD., *Toronto*
PRENTICE-HALL FRANCE, S.A.R.L., *Paris*
PRENTICE-HALL OF INDIA (PRIVATE) LTD., *New Delhi*
PRENTICE-HALL OF JAPAN, INC., *Tokyo*
PRENTICE-HALL DE MEXICO, S.A., *Mexico City*

CONTENTS

Stay Well
Every Year
of Your Life:

Dr. Molner's
Guide to Total Health

1

YOU CAN

ACHIEVE TOTAL HEALTH

MAXIM 1 *Learn the simple—and natural—rules of getting the food, liquid and oxygen you need for health.*

Naturally, you don't need a book to teach you the basic rules of staying alive. People ate, drank and breathed for thousands of years before they learned to write books, much less began to understand the *reasons* for doing what came naturally.

Unhappily, the more sophisticated society has become, the more efforts have been made by some individuals to invent fancy rules, so that they could cash in on "explaining" them to the gullible or on selling some nostrum or other. People caught up with the "medicine man" and his snake oil of years ago. Now it becomes necessary to catch up with some of the newer and less obvious catchpenny notions.

One widely voiced theory says that "we are what we eat," which is a sort of half-truth. Obviously we can't be anything that we don't (in one way or another) consume, so the notion sounds plausible.

But does it mean that we have to eat some rigidly prescribed diet for maximum health? It certainly does *not*. The Eskimo survives on the foods he can find in the Arctic. In the jungles of the tropics, populations exist at least equally well on entirely different diets. True, there are health hazards in these climates, as well as in many others, but the varieties of possible diets that are completely adequate are numberless.

You can have a fire that burns coal, wood, gas, coke, oil, peat or even buffalo chips. All the fires provide heat. In the same sense, although a bit more complicated, any number of food combinations can give us all we need for health. For a common example, most of us are aware that a serving or two of leafy green vegetables is part of a healthful diet, but whether that means spinach, Swiss chard, beet tops, lettuce, cabbage, watercress, collard greens, dandelion greens or any of a great many more doesn't make any important difference.

Within very broad limits, we find the comparatively small number of essential materials wherever we live. There are, I agree, specific areas of the globe where something may be locally lacking, but these are the exceptions. It is quite safe to say that you can select any adequate diet anywhere in the world, then find another diet, just as adequate, that contains not a single item of food in common with the other one. And you can do this again and again and again. In other words, there are many sources of every type of food that is needed for robust health.

A Lesson in Sun and Codfish

Let's take just one example of this. We all need Vitamin D. Lack of it, especially in childhood, leads to soft and, hence, irregularly formed bones—bow legs, distorted joints, structural deformities of the chest, as "pigeon breast" or "funnel chest." In short, rickets.

To avoid this risk, it is common practice to give babies cod-liver oil or similar fish-liver oils, which are rich in Vitamin D.

How, you may well ask, can this be available both in the tropics and the polar regions? What about people who live in areas where nobody ever heard of a codfish, much less its liver or Vitamin D?

The answer is that the action of ultraviolet light (sunlight!)

on any number of common food products will convert them into Vitamin D.

The fish of the sea, little exposed to sunlight, have developed the power, over ages of history, to make maximum use of such sources as they encounter. I do not know exactly how this is done. Perhaps the almost invisibly small forms of aquatic life absorb sunlight near the surface of the water, then are eaten by larger creatures of the sea. The latter, in turn, are also devoured, so that the chemical ingredients eventually reach even larger fish, which may never venture very close to the surface.

Whatever the chemical explanation, the Eskimo gets his Vitamin D from the fish he catches and eats. In the warm and sunny climates, an abundance of sunshine provides Vitamin D more directly.

When man changes his environment some compensation may be required. The example that comes most readily to mind is part of British history—the Industrial Revolution. In smoky, foggy, cavernous streets and lofts, children got little sunshine. Rickets became common. This did not occur in the open country areas where the average youngster got plenty of sun.

We found that Vitamin D, in the form of fish-liver oil, could prevent rickets among even children who got little sun. It is, I think, a fascinating example of how things as different as sunlight and fish can fill equivalent needs.

The deeper lesson is that Nature adapts. Throughout this book you will find repeated references to Nature's workings. We can, it is obvious, throw Nature off stride (as with the deprivation of sunlight), and Nature works slowly. Nature does not instantly accommodate to the artificial changes in conditions that are created by mankind. Over thousands of years, she does.

It behooves us, then, to learn as much as we can about the manner in which Nature operates. If there is a key thought in this volume, that is it.

The "Diet Supplement" Nonsense

A question that very frequently comes to me concerns commercial products called "diet supplements," usually identified (in the small print, anyway) as mixtures of vitamins and minerals.

A salesman would appear, in a store or at someone's front door or "introduced by a friend," and go into a glib spiel about why, if you wanted to be healthy, you had to use his diet supplement every day. The price, to anyone who analyzed what his product contained, was often exorbitant.

But worse, it was entirely unnecessary for anyone who was getting a fair representation of the foods available in the corner grocery store.

We shall soon present an outline of the basic foods which satisfy the needs of the human body. It won't take more than 5 minutes, I estimate, for you to get the food groupings firmly in your mind.

The United States Food and Drug Administration has been waging a quiet but persistent campaign against enterprises (often bearing imposing names) that profit by scaring people into thinking that an easily obtained, well-balanced diet isn't enough—that you must have "supplements" to be healthy. Sadly, these promoters too often go beyond the line and promise, or at least their salesmen do, that the "supplements" will prevent all sorts of diseases—from cancer to corns. The law can then step in, however, and put an end to any enterprise that preys on the gullibility of people who are overimpressed by wild promises.

I could hardly begin to list all of the variations that have been devised to sell "supplement capsules" or the like. And I certainly can't attempt to guess what some sharpshooter will devise next. The "supplements" may be harmless enough, or they may be sound mixtures of chemicals, but they aren't necessary for anyone getting a well-balanced diet.

Besides the commercial sharpshooters, there are well-intentioned individuals who grab some small fact and exaggerate it. I think that is the origin of an idea that led to quite a flurry of inquiries from readers of my newspaper column on health.

Readers began asking, and so did people with whom I came in personal contact, whether eating raw eggs was dangerous because eggs prevented absorption of biotin, one of the B-complex vitamins.

A morsel of data seems to support such a theory—unless you

look at it carefully. Raw egg white, it is true, does inhibit the absorption of biotin because egg white contains a chemical called avidin. (Cooking of the egg produces chemical changes that prevent this from happening.)

When you examine this idea scientifically, the first fact to keep in mind is that avidin does not remain in the digestive tract very long. If you eat a raw egg for breakfast, it isn't going to prevent absorption of biotin at lunch or supper. Second, we need only a fraction of a milligram of biotin a day, and we have little chance of not getting enough except under the most restricted of starvation diets.

The whole notion, in other words, amounted to building up a scare story on the basis of a small fact that was not applied or interpreted correctly.

Whether, for entirely different reasons, we may prefer not to eat raw eggs is another matter. Most of the time it is safe, but germs can, on occasion, be present; as a long-range matter of safety, I want my eggs cooked.

All sorts of diet fads are popping up constantly: the idea that cod-liver oil will lubricate arthritic joints; that vinegar, or vinegar and honey, is a medicine; that going on a diet of nothing but grapes (or some other single food) for a week will "drive the poisons out of your body"; that you shouldn't eat fish and milk at the same meal. And so on. That all of these notions are folklore is the best that can be said for them. None is necessary for health.

But how, you reasonably ask, can a person be expected to keep up-to-date enough to recognize all of the curious diet fads that gain circulation?

You can't. But if you know what constitutes a balanced diet, you have the practical knowledge necessary to eat a thoroughly healthful diet. You will be perfectly safe (and often much better off) if you ignore such odd-ball fads and whims as will, unquestionably, be offered to you.

What a Balanced Diet Is

Here is the way to judge your food, to see that you eat the right things. Simply learn the seven basic types of food. They are:

1. *Protein*   This is the building material for our bodies. There is no substitute for it. The rich sources of protein are lean meat, eggs, nuts, cheese and, to a lesser extent, other dairy products, fish and sea foods. One or two servings per day of these "protein foods" is adequate. I shall enlarge on this later.

2. *Green Vegetables*   Vegetables contain a little protein, some more than others. Their purpose in the diet is not primarily to furnish protein. Grown in the sun, these vegetables provide vegetable fibers (or roughage, if you prefer that term) that give a certain amount of bulk to our food. Through action of sun and soil, the green vegetables contain traces of both vitamins and minerals that we need—and we need no more than traces of them. One or two servings a day.

3. *Yellow Vegetables*   Squash, carrots, sweet potatoes, yams and others contain Vitamin A, which has a variety of uses—promoting good skin texture, good eye sensitivity to faint light, and good resistance to infections. A serving a day: perhaps, for example, carrots in a salad, carrot sticks or the familiar peas-and-carrots combination.

4. *Cereals*   Bread, toast, breakfast food, dishes made of oats, rye, barley or other grains. A couple of slices of bread a day and a dish of breakfast food are, for all practical purposes, enough for the average individual. Virtually all of us eat more than that. The cereals, or grains, are a good source of protein. They are also rich in carbohydrate and include traces of minerals and substantial amounts of the useful Vitamin B-1.

5. *Calcium*   By which I mean, for most adults, a glass or two of milk, or the equivalent. For children, a quart a day. Cow's milk has been called "the most complete food we have," with the exception (for babies) of mother's milk. Milk is richer in protein than most vegetables but does not rank with meat in this respect. It has some fat, some carbohydrate. One can drink skim milk and get the calcium without most of the fat. One can have a taste for cottage cheese and not have the need for milk from the standpoint of calcium.

Green vegetables can supply a good deal of calcium. But generally speaking, I still do not believe we should omit milk as a staple of diet. It has too many valuable components. We can find substitutes for its various valuable constituents, but no one substitute replaces all of them.

6. *Fresh fruits*   Vitamin C is the one great vitamin paramount in fruit, especially the citrus type, which includes oranges, grapefruit, lemons and limes. This is the reason for the widespread use of citrus juices, as well as tomato juice which also is rich in Vitamin C.

The terrible lesson about the need of Vitamin C came from British seafarers. After weeks or months at sea, living mostly on hardtack and dried beef, sailors got scurvy. Teeth fell out. Men lost their strength. There was bleeding under the skin. Sailors were easy prey for other diseases.

Although Vitamin C was not identified until long afterward, ship doctors stumbled onto a good source that could be carried on long voyages—lime juice. And scurvy was conquered.

7. *Fat and carbohydrate*   This comes last because nobody has to be watchful about getting enough of these food elements. Appetite alone is a sufficient guide. If anything, in a land where food is plentiful, we have to take care not to eat too much, because these are essentially energy foods or fuel foods, rather than building foods like protein and calcium, or regulating foods like the vitamins. If we eat more fat and carbohydrate than we need, we store the excess. In a word, we get fat.

Carbohydrates, of course, are essentially starches and sugars of which a variety exist—although this point is of scant importance to us in the ordinary choice of what we eat. Our bodies accept the carbohydrates and convert them into a usable form, blood sugar.

In this regard, a most enlightening experiment was worked out with a group of children. Some were allowed to eat all the carbohydrate they wanted—starchy and sweet foods—*before* being given protein foods. These children ate too much carbohydrate but not enough protein.

Other children were given protein *first*, then the carbohydrate foods. They automatically ate enough protein but stopped when they had enough. Then they ate moderately of carbohydrates—enough, but not too much.

In plain language, this means that we can trust our appetites if we apply common sense. We've learned over the centuries to eat our meat and vegetables first and not to spoil our appetites by filling up beforehand on starch and sugar. There is sound reason for Italians mixing meat sauces for their spaghetti; it is more than just a matter of flavor. The meat (and grated cheese) add protein to the spaghetti's carbohydrate.

You will find similar rational patterns running through the widely differing forms of cooking in different parts of the world.

What about Vegetarian Diets?

You might even ask me about vegetarianism—which I regard as an artificial diet and, hence, a fad, but it is one that also has pretty much bowed to the realities. I have no objection to vegetarianism for those who happen to care for it and follow it with a certain amount of logic.

The average man, it has been calculated, would have to cram down his gullet something like 30 pounds of vegetables and fruit a day to get the nutrition he needs. Although vegetable products contain a little protein and vegetable fat, and some (such as grains and raisins) are quite rich in carbohydrate, a lamb chop, for example, has about 15 times as much protein content as an equal weight of banana. Nuts are also rich in protein, carbohydrate and vegetable fat.

In practice, the vegetarians usually take care of their need for protein by eating eggs, nuts, milk and cheese. These, with the exception of nuts, are not vegetable products. They are from animal sources. The combination can furnish a very adequate diet—but it isn't purely vegetarian!

The essential point I want to make is simply this: There is nothing rigid about a balanced diet. It can vary enormously from north to south and east to west, depending on what kinds of foods are plentiful and what people like.

Knowing the seven basic kinds of food, as listed above, gives anyone the information he needs. A serving or two of each kind each day will provide the protein we need, the fat and the carbohydrate. All the necessary vitamins will be supplied, as will all of the minerals we need—calcium, iron, phosphorus, potassium, sodium, copper, manganese and so on (of some we need only faint traces).

The one exception is that, in some parts of the world (and the American Midwest is an example) there is a paucity of iodine. The amount we need was once described as "about as much as you would get by smelling the stopper of an iodine bottle once a day." That's what we mean by a "trace."

Lack of iodine, we learned in the 1920's, was the cause of goiter. The thyroid gland needs a trace of iodine. If it is lacking, the gland begins to enlarge, trying to make up by sheer size what it lacks in efficiency. This enlargement is a "goiter." The answer was quite simple: adding a trifling amount of iodine in the form of potassium iodide to ordinary table salt. Its use brought an end to most goiter trouble.

It might well be that we would have less goiter today even without the iodization of salt. Why? Because sea food of all kinds is rich in iodine. Forty years ago we couldn't walk into a supermarket in the Midwest and find shrimp and oysters. Except for dried or smoked fish, the iodine-rich fish from the ocean were eaten only by people living near the seacoast. The fresh-water inland fish lacked the iodine. Modern marketing and transportation are a distinct aid to health. We can buy citrus fruit at any time of year, 2,000 miles from where it is grown. Freezing processes give us vegetables the year 'round, instead of limiting us to potatoes, cabbage, dried beans and the like in winter.

The balanced diet is easy, now. Tinkering with fads is an indoor pastime that seems to appeal to quite a lot of people, but it isn't necessary for health.

You might also ask, "If a balanced diet includes all the necessary vitamins and minerals, is there really any need for vitamin capsules and 'food supplements'?"

The answer is simple. No. For infants, Vitamin D is an excellent precaution until the baby has grown up enough to have a suitable variety of foods. After that, the balanced diet will, indeed, fulfill our needs.

If the diet, over some period of time, becomes persistently off balance, then the need for vitamins from some other source begins to appear. The "meat-and-potatoes-and-pie eater," who has been brought up disliking vegetables and fruits, is the sort of person who is inviting trouble for himself. For him, a daily capsule of mixed vitamins is useful. But he'd still be better off learning to eat the simple balanced diet.

Food faddists, in my experience, are often neurotic, or are people with health problems they hope to overcome by trick diets or gullible people who have been scared into believing some of the claptrap. The people of rugged health (and sensible eating habits) just go about their business, eating the normal balanced diets that keep them healthy.

No, in ordinary life, ordinary good sense and a simple understanding of proper eating is all we need.

In later life, however, the picture can be different. Hospitals have learned that the old, enfeebled patient who is brought in suffering from malnutrition and the manifold conditions that spring from it is so often starved for vitamins that it isn't a bad idea to give every such patient immediate doses of vitamins.

The reason, however, is not that the balanced diet has failed these people. Instead, it is that they have long ceased to follow a balanced diet—if, indeed, they ever did!

PROBLEMS OF THE OLDER PERSON

The old person, and particularly the old person living alone, in too many instances gradually changes eating habits. It's "too much trouble" to keep on cooking regular meals that provide suitable variety. Cooking just for oneself instead of for a family lacks zest. A bunch of radishes that adds a fillip to a family meal becomes quite a different matter when one person says, "So I'll have to eat radishes every day for a week if I'm to use up the bunch."

It is easy to slide into the habit of cooking some sort of casserole dish that will do for the main part of dinner several days in a row. It's as much effort to cook enough greens for one person as to cook them for ten.

Oh, it's not hard to understand and to sympathize with the

person, getting on in years, who changes eating habits. It seems so much easier to "open a can of tuna," or "just have some beans," than to remain true to former eating habits. Sometimes teeth no longer are good enough to make meat as pleasurable to eat. There's the constant temptation to settle for a sandwich and a cup of tea.

I regret to say that I have no ready solution for this sort of problem. Such activities as "Meals on Wheels" are a blessed boon for some of these old people. Homes for old people are learning to pay shrewd heed to meals that are attractive as well as composed of the basic foods. I have heard, here and there, of groups of older people who take turns preparing good meals for each other instead of subsisting on the snacks they would prepare for themselves if eating alone. Sweden is developing an organization of visiting helpers for its old people—helpers who may do anything from grocery shopping to cooking to housekeeping.

Ingenuity can solve the problem in different ways. Sometimes economics makes it more difficult. It is nice to be able to afford to go out to restaurants several times a week, but not everybody can. But realizing that this is one of the large problems of growing old is the first step toward solving it. Every one of us should remember and avoid this pitfall.

Nutrition could be the subject of an entire book, if we were to go into even a few of the ramifications of food chemistry. My point is that this isn't necessary. I am sure that any careful reader now has the fundamentals in mind. Eating—and eating properly —is a basic rule of health.

So, too, is liquid intake. Water, indeed, is a more critical need than food, since a person can survive only about a week (11 days is the longest known time) without water but can exist several times as long without food.

THIRST—A GOOD REGULATOR

The mechanism of thirst is a good enough control for most of us. There is, technically, such a thing as getting too much water, but it happens only under abnormal conditions. We're talking about health, not sickness, and our ordinary tendency is to drink too little water.

Without getting into a long thesis, let's remind ourselves briefly of the uses of water. The body is 70 percent or more water; the blood, 90 percent water. We need water to convert our food into a liquid form that will move readily through our digestive organs.

We use water to keep our bodies cool (perspiration). Water is necessary to carry away the waste matter from our bodies. We even exhale water. In 24 hours this amounts to a substantial quantity of fluid. If you doubt it, just pause to remember that when you breathe on your glasses to clean them, a single breath permits a visible amount of moisture to condense!

The rule of thumb is that we need about 6 pints of water a day, on the average, and considerably more in hot weather or when exertion makes us sweat. But oddly enough, the person working under such conditions of heat and exertion is rarely the person who suffers from insufficient fluid intake. He gets thirsty and drinks a lot of water!

Rather, it is usually the inactive individual—the quiet person, the invalid or the older person—whose water intake is insufficient.

We do not have to drink anything like 6 pints of water as such. Some of it is in the form of milk, tea, coffee or other beverages. Or in soup. Or salad—leafy vegetables can be more than 90 percent water, an apple or an orange 85 percent or more. Such a substantial item as an egg is about 74 percent water, and beef is more than 60 percent water.

We constantly are pumping a quart of blood a minute through our kidneys, filtering out impurities molecule by molecule and particle by particle.

Have we said enough to present a convincing argument that a sufficient intake of water, in one form or another, is important?

When we get too little water, the body automatically tries to conserve what it has. Less water will be used to carry off the wastes filtered out by the kidneys. The urine thus will be less diluted. In a person with a tendency toward kidney stones, this will intensify the trouble. On the other hand, drinking plenty of fluids will keep the urine diluted, and the salts which otherwise might form into stones will wash away. This is not something that will make a discernible difference in days or weeks; in a matter of months or years it can.

For another example, take constipation. It has been a revelation to me to discover, through letters from newspaper readers, how many people never realize the importance of water in bowel action. It is very well understood, by doctors and nurses, especially those caring for elderly patients.

An invalid, along in years, requires less energy food than a robust, hard-working young adult. Appetite is likely to be poor. The patient eats sparingly of foods that satisfy hunger most easily but lacks the brisk urge to eat foods containing "roughage" —vegetables and fruits with the cellulose fibers, which are of little if any nourishment value but provide bulk.

The result is the accumulation of relatively little waste in the bowel. Until enough has accumulated, there is little or no urge for the bowel to move. The waste matter dries and hardens; constipation presently reaches serious proportions.

We are lucky enough to have a medication, dioctyl sodium sulfosuccinate, a softening agent, which does wonders in easing this sort of trouble, but that's a matter of correcting the trouble after it has occurred. Why not learn the lesson and put it to good use sooner? The answer: moisture!

Many times have I received letters like this: "I had been troubled with constipation for 30 years, but after your comment that I should drink more water, I decided to try it. Since then I have been drinking two glasses of water a day, and I've found that it cleared up my trouble. I had no idea that it was so simple."

This is one of the things that every doctor knows, but he has trouble communicating this knowledge to people who don't really believe that simple remedies can be important. For whatever reason, people seem to want the doctor to give them something complicated, something mysterious, abstruse or medicinal. They don't want simple, inexpensive answers from the doctor.

Maybe we physicians have been at fault in not trying in the right way (the use of plain language) to overcome this peculiarity. If so, all I can say is that I'm doing my best to tell people of easy, inexpensive measures and to teach them to recognize the problems that cannot be met with nostrums but demand skilled, experienced treatment.

Anyway, a couple of glasses of water a day, the most inexpensive remedy I know, is an extremely effective solution for a very large number of people who complain of constipation. It helps avoid kidney stones for some. It is a sensible health precaution that generally helps keep our physical equipment in good working condition. Because it is so simple and, for the most part, does its good work so slowly, people really see its value only in special instances.

That is why I consider it important enough to include among the first rules of health.

LET'S THINK ABOUT OUR BREATHING

Finally, let's devote a few words to breathing. "Sure," you say. "I breathe all the time." Of course you do. If you stop breathing, you die. But *how* do you breathe?

Now please, *please* do not start anticipating some strange, secret way of breathing that is better than any other way. Again, I'm not going to offer some "secret" method that improves on the way Julius Caesar or the original Fred Flintstone used to breathe. Nothing of the sort.

I'm only going to call attention to a long-established but little-known fact about how our lungs work. The lungs are empty cavities. We draw air in, we expel it. The fresh air puts oxygen into the blood that courses through numerous blood vessels in the lungs. The blood then picks up carbon dioxide thrown off by the blood, and we breathe that out.

But where does this exchange of oxygen and carbon dioxide take place?

Why, on the inner surface of the lung tissue!

The lungs are not a couple of smooth little penny balloons. The entire inner surface is a network of tubes that branch off into smaller tubes, thence into clusters of little sacs called alveoli. The total surface of all these little sacs is enormous—something like

100 square yards, or perhaps 30 times the total surface of the outside of the body.

It is entirely possible, or probable or, in fact, unavoidable that some of the air we draw into our lungs never comes in contact with the surfaces of the alveoli. It never does any good. We breathe it in—and we breathe it out again as fresh as it originally was. Indeed, if it weren't for that small fact, there wouldn't be a great deal of point in trying such things as mouth-to-mouth respiration in cases of drowning or other disastrous accidents. There would be no point in forcing spent or used-up air into the victim's lungs. But it isn't all used up. We use, with each breath, only the oxygen of those particles that reach the tissue surfaces of the lungs.

At this point you are beginning to ask, "All right, so what do I *do* about it?"

I can give you my answer in a milk bottle. You've rinsed bottles. You know how the film of milk clings to the glass a little bit. Fill the bottle gently, and pour the water out again gently; some of the film remains on the glass. Then what do you do?

Why, you fill the bottle again, and you shake it. The water sloshes around, and each molecule of water, as it bumps against the milk-filmed surface, picks up and carries away its particle of milk. A couple of good sloshes does more good than five or six placid fillings and dumpings.

It's the same with air in the lungs. I'm not a special devotee of "deep breathing," which is supposed to expand the upper part of the lungs, or of "belly breathing," which is supposed to put the lower parts of the lungs to work. I'm just an advocate of the "sloshing technique."

When you happen to think of it, take an extra-deep breath. Or make a noisy, breezy, extra-hard exhalation. It's very little different from sloshing the rinse water around in the milk bottle.

When our small fry run, jump and holler, they are doing a mighty good job of "air sloshing" in their lungs. When a baby does some unexplained bellowing, or his daddy spends an afternoon walking around and occasionally swinging a golf club to hit a little ball, or throwing a much larger ball to hit some tenpins, or pushing a lawn mower or painting the kitchen ceiling (which keeps his arms moving), the air swirls beneficially in the lungs.

You can sit in a rocking chair on the porch of the most expensive resort hotel in the world, surrounded by the freshest air in the world, but if you placidly breathe in and breathe out, you aren't going to get the same benefits that are enjoyed by us ordinary people who have to breathe ordinary air but keep the air swirling as we breathe it.

At this point you may be saying to yourself, "Well, just what did Dr. Molner tell me, except that some exercise is a good thing?" That's just about it!

All of us have moments when we think "a breath of fresh air is what I need." Fine! Get it! But don't assume that just breathing some air on the front porch is necessarily better than the air you've been breathing indoors. Get some activity. It's important to you. Why does a tired athlete gulp air? Because, automatically, he breathes gustily to send the air swirling into as many as possible of the countless alveoli of his lungs.

I don't want you to waste time trying to memorize anything in this chapter—unless perhaps, in the most condensed fashion possible, the list of seven basic foods. Just read and you'll remember the general ideas.

Don't bother trying to remember that the little air sacs in the lungs are called alveoli. That's not important. But keep in mind that some activity, some gusty breathing when you feel logey, is a good way to help your breathing. Simple? Certainly. But some of the basic rules of health are just that simple.

2

DON'T JUST STAND THERE

MAXIM 2 *Exercise is one of the necessities of life.*

Oddly, we give it very little thought. It doesn't need a great deal, I grant, but it does need some.

How much do your friends know about exercise? If you pin them down, you often find that they know almost nothing about it. "Exercise is healthful," they may say. Or, "It's good for you and helps your appetite." Or, "It aids the circulation."

Some, fruitfully influenced by such people as Dr. Paul Dudley White, may remark on the value of exercise in retarding hardening of the arteries. But few people, in my experience, even bother to wonder why or how exercise is useful. It is more than useful. It is necessary.

Curiously, there is a widespread belief that certain exercises have curative powers. The three most frequent questions I encounter in letters received through my newspaper column are: "What diet should I follow for my condition?" "What vitamins should I take?" "What exercises will help my trouble?"

All three questions are based on a greatly distorted view of how to care for the human body or cure its ills. All have a place, but expecting them to be cures is true only in certain limited circumstances.

There is a difference, of course, between exercises and exercise. Let's talk about the latter.

Exercise does, indeed, "help the circulation," but in a subtler way than many realize. Circulation is more than a matter of the heart forcing blood through the arteries and then back to the heart via the veins.

As the arteries branch out through the body into smaller and smaller sizes, they ultimately extend into capillaries, so small that they carry particles of microscopic dimensions. Then occurs what we might call a "seepage," although there are more technical terms for it. Oxygen and nutrients diffuse through the walls of the capillaries and are carried by a liquid known as "tissue fluid" to the countless cells that make up the body.

This tissue fluid does not return the way it came. Instead, it finds its way into lymph ducts, through lymph nodes which filter out impurities, and ultimately back to the blood stream again.

Since it carries large numbers of white blood cells, this lymphatic system is an important barrier against disease. The white cells attack and destroy bacteria. The residue of this valuable, invisible biological warfare is part of the material filtered out by the lymph nodes.

Besides carrying nutrients, carting away discarded refuse from the tissues and doing battle with bacteria, the lymphatic system also plays a part in transporting fats from the digestive system to the blood stream, but there's no point in going into all its precise functions. Obviously the lymphatic system is of basic importance.

But what causes the tissue fluid (called lymph after it reaches the ducts) to flow along? Why, the massaging action of the organs and tissues around the ducts!

This does not mean that you have to be physically active for this to happen. Even the pulsation of blood through the veins helps, since infinitely small lymph networks are woven closely around the veins.

Every movement of the body, whether it is the heartbeat, the movement of the breathing lungs, the automatic motion of the intestines or any other, does its part in promoting the lymph flow.

More vigorous activity naturally adds its help.

Now let's talk about the flow in the veins. Here again exercise helps, although to a different degree. Blood flowing back to the heart is propelled principally by the force of heart action, but it is also aided by muscular activity.

Since the most difficult flow is from the feet and legs, since they are farthest from the heart and, in addition, the blood has to be lifted the entire distance, let's think for a minute about the veins there. (This will be of importance later on when we discuss the common problem of varicose veins.)

The veins in the legs are equipped with a great many valves that permit the blood to flow in only one direction: toward the heart. With each pulse, some blood is forced upward, opening the valves by its upward surge. When that pulse ends, the valves are forced shut again by the weight of the blood above them.

Where does the "exercise" come in? In two ways. But first of all remember that the veins are soft, pliable tissue, with nothing to support them except the flesh around them. If this flesh is firm and strong, it gives good support. If it is weak and flabby, and the muscles have lost their tone, the veins do not have the support they need. The veins sag or bulge, the little valves may be pulled somewhat out of shape and be unable to open and close as efficiently as they should. The circulation, resultingly, begins to suffer. There may or may not be varicose veins, but that isn't our immediate question. Circulation is, to some slight degree at least, impaired. (That's why elastic stockings help in such cases.)

Now for the second point. Movement of the many muscles in the legs, just by steady tensing and relaxing, helps squeeze the blood upward.

If you think this is minor, you should talk to some of the people whose faulty circulation has been helped by a very simple bit of advice. When circulation is too slow in the legs and feet, the muscles start to protest. They start cramping.

Therefore, people who have some circulatory impairment, particularly if they have jobs requiring them to be on their feet much of the time, are logical candidates for foot and leg cramps. This applies more to the person who stands still than to the person who has to do a great deal of walking. The letter carrier who spends hours walking may, if he isn't careful, develop foot troubles, but the clerk who stands at a window all day long, selling stamps, may have more trouble with cramps!

For such complaints, therefore, we urge the individual to change position often, to walk around—even if he can pace no more than two or three steps. If you have a stool to sit on, hook your toes around it in different positions. Even such a little thing as wiggling your toes inside your shoes can help. If you want to try a small experiment, put your hand on the calf of your leg or on the side of the leg. Then wiggle your toes. You will feel the leg muscles moving.

People are sometimes greatly astonished to find out how much relief they gain from such simple "exercises," but when the "why" of it is understood, it no longer is so astonishing. It's just good sense.

Although I've applied this to the feet and legs, because circulation is most likely to be importantly impaired there, the same factors exist elsewhere in the body.

Exercise *does* help the circulation, and beyond the common idea that it helps only by speeding up the heart to send blood coursing more abundantly through the arteries. It does that, too, of course, but that isn't the point I want to make. I want you to have an understanding of the way very simple, mild exercise can benefit you.

I don't insist that everybody be a weight-lifter, or run two miles before breakfast, or spend so many hours daily or weekly doing push-ups or using a rowing machine or whatever other strenuous exercise may be favored by some enthusiasts. But moderate, regular exercise is good for all of us. We don't have to do violent setting-up exercises or exhaust ourselves trying to be modern Tarzans.

Ride a bike. Dig in the garden. Pull weeds. Bowl. Do a few calisthenics if that's your preference. A rocking chair is better than the kind of overstuffed chair you snooze in—if you rock. It keeps your muscles moving a bit. In fact, you may recall that a "rocking bed" (one which tips back and forth from head to foot) was invented to help the circulation of paralyzed people.

You don't have to go in for anything that costs a lot of money, you don't have to learn special kinds of exercises. Just keep yourself moving, and you are genuinely doing something for your health.

As to the strenuous forms of exercise, I certainly have no objection to them—if (and this is a big IF) you enjoy them and engage in them regularly. But there is little benefit and considerable risk in trying to be a "week-end athlete"—sitting at a desk all week long and then trying to make up for it by an overdose of exertion Saturday afternoon. If you huff and puff and feel pretty tired after playing 36 (or 18) holes of golf once a week or once a month, you aren't helping yourself. You'd do better to play half as much golf twice as often, and you'd do even better by finding some way of getting a modest amount of exercise every day.

Now that you have some specific reasons—although there are others which I shall discuss, and they are important, too—you can fit the fundamental facts into some of the situations which occur time after time. Or used to.

Many of you certainly recall the days when, for an elderly person, a broken hip was close to being a sentence of death. Old bones knit slowly. The broken hip meant keeping the patient flat in bed, with the least possible movement.

With a broken arm, or leg, or shoulder or ribs it was possible to use casts or tape and let the patient move about or, at least, sit up. But not with a broken hip.

The hip itself was not fatal. Instead, some rather common infection got a start. Usually it was pneumonia. The body, without the benefit of exercise, quickly lost its defensive ability. Sluggish circulation ensued. Death generally followed. The broken hip was only indirectly the disaster. The long, enforced immobility was the deadly factor, because it crippled the defenses.

To a lesser extent, extended bed rest illustrates the same factors at work. How shaky you are when you first try to walk after a long period of invalidism!

This, however, is primarily a matter of loss of muscle tone. With disuse, the muscles soon begin to lose their strength. Although of significance, this is not as serious as the almost total lack of movement that used to be necessary for the broken-hip patient, who couldn't move at all without pain or danger of interfering with the healing of the hip. Other patients can use their arms with quite some freedom as a rule, can wiggle their toes, flex their knees, roll from side to side or be carefully turned.

These days, as you doubtless know, the patient with the broken hip usually recovers instead of dying. The difference is the process of "pinning" the hip with metal "nails" so the patient can safely move to some degree almost at once. True, this requires an operation, but the risks of surgery are trivial compared to the very nearly certain tragedy that the fracture otherwise meant to the aged.

And there is a third example that most assuredly needs to be emphasized.

Back in the 1930's it was the accepted practice to keep a patient immobilized in bed after any surgery except the most minor. A week or 10 days was routine after surgery for a faulty appendix. About the same time was expected after childbirth. It was taken for granted that such a period (and longer for more severe cases) was necessary to allow incisions to heal and to permit the patient to regain his strength.

Then one day in a Detroit hospital an energetic (and obviously free-thinking) patient had his appendix out. He said he wanted to get up—and was automatically shushed by nurses and doctors. Oh yes! Doctors have been victims of popular misconceptions, too! We all have our blind spots. We all are guilty of accepting as "true" the things we have become accustomed to believe.

But in this case the patient refused to accept the "No-No" response that was then universal. The day after the operation one of the nurses saw him nonchalantly wandering down the corridor!

Horrified, she insisted that he get back to bed before something disastrous happened to him; she then called his doctor.

Happily for medical progress, the doctor was willing to listen to his patient's argument and willing to look facts in the face. Not only did the early-after-surgery activity fail to harm this patient, but it seemed to help him, for he was able to go home in remarkably short time.

The doctor began to wonder. He tried getting some other

patients up a little earlier. They did well. He tried others still earlier and found that they progressed even better.

This was the beginning of "early ambulation." It is to me interesting, but a matter of no great pride, that when the doctor reported his findings to other doctors at a meeting, some stiff-necked individuals refused to listen to him; one even threatened to denounce him publicly if he did not give up his ideas at once.

In what happened after that history gives me much more reason for pride. Thinking doctors were in the vast majority. They examined the evidence and acted on the facts. The stiff-necks soon had to admit that the new idea was right.

Today it is quite usual for a patient, even after such a serious operation as open-heart surgery, to sit up within a day or two and be on his feet (however briefly) in another day.

Sutures applied with the skill that any surgeon must have are as strong as healthy flesh itself. Unless the patient's tissues are extraordinarily weak (which can occur with some few diseases), he is in no danger of "breaking open the incision." That just does not happen.

But he cannot lie abed for a week and not suffer the consequences of inactivity. Call it "moving around," or call it "exercise," or call it what you wish, but early ambulation is now one of the cardinal rules of restoring patients to health after surgery.

Occasionally, patients resent it or doubt their ability to comply. They are physically tired and emotionally overwrought after their operations. With this I can sympathize. I've had an operation or two myself. We have a natural instinct to say, "Look, I've been through some serious surgery. I'm tired. I want to lie still and regain my strength before I start gallivanting around."

The mother who has had a baby looks forward to a week or so of lying quietly and having somebody else do the work and the running. I haven't been a mother myself, but my patient wife Mary, has had two babies, and I think I can faintly guess the attitude.

But I know what experience has revealed to us, and (my apologies to the natural feelings of all women who have gone through the travail of childbirth) I know that getting up and moving around early is the best insurance for rapid recovery of full health.

Physical activity is, beyond any shadow of doubt, truly important to vigorous physical health.

You've doubtless noticed that I haven't said anything about hard exercise. I don't think it is necessarily required, especially by adults. It depends on what you are accustomed to. You don't have to be a football player or weight-lifter to be healthy.

Rather, in my opinion, the key word (or key thought) is *brisk*. And this will vary somewhat, depending upon your age.

For children, the usual activities and antics are natural and right. The infant creeps. The toddler toddles. In fact, if he's healthy and normal, he toddles so much that we wonder where he gets all his energy.

As a small boy he wrestles, climbs trees, roller-skates, plays tag, begins to play baseball, hockey or whatever the prevailing sport is. Or he ought to. This is the sort of activity that gets him out into the fresh air and sunshine, keeps his muscles in good tone, develops his lungs, helps build good posture. It is part of growing up.

Comparative physical fitness tests already have shown that too much riding to school and not enough walking, too much sitting in front of television and not enough vigorous play, has had an inevitably softening effect on young Americans.

I'm quite aware that some people have resented the disclosure of these facts and tried to deny them. They point to some of our outstanding athletes as proof of their denial. The argument doesn't wash. The fact that some—indeed, quite a lot—of our children get plenty of exercise does not by any means indicate that all do. The presence of 50,000 people in a stadium watching the performance of a few trained athletes doesn't make athletes of the 50,000.

By personal observation, and comparing muscle-performance tests of our own and foreign children, I can come to no conclusion except that, in general, we ought to lay down a few simple rules in the home to keep the small fry from doing too much sitting.

I certainly have no objection to TV as such, any more than I object to ice cream cones, pie or time for play. I *do* object to letting any of these things get out of hand. Enough is enough.

Television should be regarded as a treat, not a steady diet.

My notion of the way to handle the matter would be to allow a child, say, one program a day, and to limit the choice to programs late in the afternoon or early in the evening. That is when a normally active child might very well start quieting down. From the TV programming that I've noted, I gather that the TV people have, to some useful extent, taken this into consideration and chosen suitable times for children's programs. It's up to parents to make sure that the youngsters don't come home from school and plop down in front of some wheezy B movie. That's the time of day that should be spent in riding bikes, playing ball and getting air, sun and exercise. And remember, you can't feed a child too much sweets for several years, then expect to change things without a protest. It is the same with TV.

Now, you may feel that we've gotten somewhat away from our topic, but I don't think so. The early attitude toward exercise is one which, like any other habit, is pretty likely to follow through life. The sit-still child becomes a sit-still teen ager, a too-plump young adult and a rump-sprung old one.

The person who grows up getting plenty of exercise usually misses it if it is shut off later. Whether it's sailing a boat, hiking, bowling, swimming, handball, golf, paddling a canoe or spading the garden, some form of exercise should be consciously adopted as a person outgrows the roistering pursuits of youth. Daily calisthenics are fine if your preference lies that way—but don't think that two minutes of gentle arm-waving once a week is going to be much good.

Quite often I am asked, "What is the best exercise?" I could correctly say that there isn't any "best" exercise, but the most universally available one is walking. Not strolling but *walking*. Remember that word *brisk*. At 70 a brisk walk isn't the same as at 17, but your common sense will be a perfectly adequate guide, so long as you keep that key word in mind and genuinely try to abide by it.

I know one man who had a city job and regularly walked home from work, a matter of about 6 miles. The last time I saw him he was retired, but he was lean, alert and happy.

Not everyone can spend that amount of time in walking, but

everyone, if he uses even a little ingenuity, can find some way of getting exercise. There's an important business executive, for example, who rises half an hour early in the morning and rides a bicycle.

If you can afford to belong to a club with a swimming pool, that's fine. But you can chin yourself on a door casing, do push-ups on the floor, play tennis in a public park, chop wood if you live in a small town. But make daily exercise a habit. Being a week-end exerciser and feeling virtuous the other 6 days a week is no substitute.

Two more facets of exercise remain. One is the matter of weight. Since we'll discuss that in detail in other chapters, I won't belabor the issue now, except to point out that only rarely is the regular exercise-taker too fat.

The other topic is cholesterol, of which so much has been said, and repeated, and mouthed, and mumbled and jumbled.

How much cholesterol has to do with hardening of the arteries is something which, at this writing, has not been specifically proved. I am more than willing to stick my neck out and assert flatly that cholesterol is certainly only one of a whole group of factors, some known, some perhaps not even suspected yet.

Tinkering with diet may have some effect on the arteries, but it is disgracefully sloppy thinking to feel that you have done something wonderful in behalf of your health merely by spreading something different on your bread or swapping salad dressings. It's not far ahead of the thinking demonstrated in the old anecdote about the backwoods family, warned about germs, announcing proudly, "Oh, we already got us a sanitary drinking cup, and everybody in the family uses it!"

Remember, I do not say that some attention to cholesterol in the diet is not warranted, but it's only a modest part of the problem.

Meanwhile we do know, from experiments that have been tried and tested repeatedly, that the amount of cholesterol circulating in the blood is most decidedly influenced by exercise. Take a group of middle-aged business men, measure their cholesterol levels, then put half of the men into a simple fitness program that requires an hour's exercise a day. Or even half that much—

but make it regular. Let the rest of them continue their usual sedentary habits.

Measure the cholesterol levels in another month or two; the active men often show a decided decrease.

Why, I continue to ask myself, do so many people spend so much time, money and worry over the amount of cholesterol in their food, when they could be shedding excess cholesterol more surely and sensibly by daily exercise?

Is it because we put an unreasonably high premium on some "easy" way? Because we refuse to honor anything that sounds simple? Because we are sheep, following whatever fad happens to appear in front of us? Because we feel that if we spend our hard-earned money for something, it necessarily has to be better than something we can have for no cost?

I'm sure I don't know the answer. But I do know that exercise is one way of lowering cholesterol levels, and I question if a more effective method exists. And I know that the exercise, at the same time, will be contributing to the health not only of your arteries but of your body processes generally.

Exercise is truly one of the foundations of good health. It doesn't have to be violent. It doesn't have to be of some particular type. But it should become a fixed, daily habit, and I wonder whether, when you began this chapter, you realized some of the quiet, subtle ways in which exercise protects us.

3

THE ONLY WAY TO DIET

Maxim 3 *Obesity can kill you.*

This is not hyperbole. Obesity can kill. Obesity does kill. By this time, most people are aware that fat is a health hazard, but they don't, I've found out, usually understand why.

We'll get to that. We'll also, a little later in this chapter, get around to explaining the meaning of the chapter title. It would, I am convinced, be a good thing if we abolished "diet" or "reducing diet" from the vocabulary. I think you will agree with me, after I tell you my reasons, that we would be better off if we changed our thinking, changed our viewpoint and stopped accepting the popular notion that "going on a diet" is the way to reduce. But let's take first things first.

How do we know that obesity is deadly? We have the most hard-headed evidence conceivable, the experience of life insurance companies. For them, it comes down to a matter of dollars and cents. Life-insurance rates (like any insurance rates) are based on actuarial figures, which present the picture as it actually is.

Do fat people die sooner than thin ones? Yes, indeed they do. The fatter they are, the sooner they die. This the insurance com-

38

panies know, and for the substantially overweight applicant, the insurance rate is higher (if, indeed, an extremely obese person can get insurance at all).

To me, the sheer question of how long we live is not the most important question. A long, bored, unproductive life does not balance up, in my thinking, with a shorter life that is full of interest, happiness and usefulness.

In the matter of obesity, excess fat not only shortens life but it impairs health in general (else it would not hasten death). It certainly takes its toll in happiness and usefulness.

For the person who is 50 pounds overweight, the risk of death is something like 300 percent higher at a given age than for the person of normal weight. The insurance companies can give you elaborate and impressive tables of figures showing how the death rate increases as each few extra pounds is added.

It is estimated (and I think conservatively) that one American in five is obese. Other estimates state that as high as half of the population is overweight.

Of course a few extra pounds don't matter much, if really only a few. Three, four or five. However, in blunt language, overweight is one of the things we lie about. We use words like *buxom, plump* or *stout* when we would accomplish more by saying what we mean. *Fat!*

The United States is a land of abundance. Nutritious foods and a minimum of exercise—we have the makings of overweight.

Can we blame heredity for some of it? Some authorities think so, to some degree. Others think not. Most assuredly, body builds are inherited to the extent that some of us are naturally tall and others are not. Whether we are light-boned or heavy-boned is decreed by heredity.

It is my opinion that heredity has something to do with the rate at which we metabolize food, and hence has some influence on obesity. Note that I say "some influence." I do not say it is the cause of obesity. Some people can eat more than others can without taking on excess weight. However, I doubt whether this is ever more than a mere added influence. The basic, important considerations are, first, how much we eat, and second, how much we exercise.

Dr. Jean Mayer, the Harvard nutritionist, points out that 80 percent of the children of two obese parents will be obese, too; if only one parent, 40 percent; if neither parent is obese, the children become obese only about 7 percent of the time.

How much of this is really heredity? Perhaps very little. Most of it depends on habit. The child grows up eating large meals because he sees his parents do so. Perhaps even more important, he grows up accustomed to eating high-calorie foods: cream soups, fried food, rich desserts, large amounts of starchy food. Very often he grows up having extra snacks thrust upon him— sandwiches, candy, soft drinks (and they, laden with sugar, are fattening!), a piece of pie or cake, instead of an apple, when he gets home from school.

He gets food as a reward. He gets food as consolation when he has troubles. He resorts to food when he is lonesome, bored or unhappy. It is thrust upon him; he naturally assumes that it is natural. It is no wonder that people who have been fat all their lives find it difficult to conform to a habit of eating less. They feel, understandably, that they are being "starved" if they have to eat less than they used to. Most of us can remember the "fat boy" in the neighborhood, who seemed to be perpetually eating. He didn't do it on purpose, he didn't do it because he wanted to be fat, he just did it because it was what he had learned to do.

Most of us also are familiar with the obese person who complains, "I don't eat enough to keep a bird alive, but everything I eat turns to fat." She thinks she is telling the truth, but she just doesn't realize how much she is eating. She is used to "tasting" in the kitchen, and sometimes these tastes can mean 25 or 50 calories each. She is used to having candy in the house, and a 100-calorie dip into the box is so natural for her that she doesn't realize she is doing it.

The fact is that fat people *like* to eat, which is just another way of saying that people who like to eat, and do, get fat. Did you ever know a fat person who *didn't* like to eat?

Two people—watch this sometime and see—can order exactly the same meal in a restaurant, but one will out-eat the other by a hundred or several hundred calories. One eats a lot of crackers with his soup. The other doesn't. One nibbles a stalk of celery.

The other puts away all the olives in sight. One eats part of a roll and leaves the rest of it. The other has three slices of bread and asks for extra butter. It is the accumulation of these small items, repeated day after day and year after year, that makes a person fat. That and exercise habits. The fat person may say, "But I work as hard as anybody else," and this can be true. But who scoots up and down stairs, and who goes at a deliberate pace? You know the answer. You know whether it is the thin person or the fat one that is inclined to "think on his feet," and get up and pace the floor while trying to work out some problem. And you know who is more inclined to sit still and think.

It may burn up no more than a few calories to pace the floor for a few minutes. It may represent a similarly insignificant number of calories in a trip upstairs and back, but it is most undeniably true that going quickly uses more energy than going slowly, as surely as running requires more energy than walking, and walking more than sitting.

Now, before you go jumping to the conclusion that I'm recommending that obese people rely on exercise to get rid of their extra weight, let me say that I'm not. Indeed, in the older and seriously overweight person, there are good reasons why heavy exercise should not be a substantial part of the reducing regimen. The too-heavy person can put undue strain on his heart. He can acquire any number of muscular pains, and even broken bones, from trying to switch from his accustomed habits to a vigorously athletic life. Above all, he cannot, in any event, expect exercise alone to dispose of all the fat he has been storing around his midriff for the preceding 10, 20 or 50 years. Exercise within reasonable limits, yes, by all means, and for purposes other than purely the matter of reducing. But in the final analysis, he is going to have to take weight off and then keep it off by reversing the process that put the weight on. He must learn the habit of eating less.

As he loses weight he is going to find exercise easier, and he can gradually add a second healthful habit: regular exercise.

However, we've skipped over one of the important parts of the discussion. Why is overweight harmful?

Excess fat doesn't all show. Some of it does: the double chin, the beefy thighs, the hips that mar appearance and the cut of our clothes, the bulgy tummy. While this visible fat is harmful to some degree, it is not the whole story. Fat also accumulates inside the body, unseen. It can crowd the heart and accumulate around the intestines to a degree that actually increases the pressure within the abdomen. Both the visible and invisible fat increase the work of the heart. Because of this demand and in spite of the crowding of the fat around the heart itself, enlargement of the heart can occur.

An increase in blood pressure occurs in the "lung circuit" (in which the heart accepts blood from the veins, pumps it to the lungs to acquire oxygen, then brings it back to the heart to be pumped to the rest of the body). There can and very often does occur an increase in the general blood pressure.

Shortness of breath, lethargy, swelling and disorders of the joints, pancreas and liver are common consequences.

The strain on the bony structure of the body is increased. The results become apparent with time. The hips, knees and ankles, which carry our weight, show signs of the strain over the years. The joints suffer. The edges of the bones at the pressure-bearing parts of the joints thicken. The cartilage, which is the "padding" in the joints, is hammered down thinner. The joints become creaky and painful. It is often called "arthritis" but that isn't the best name for it. The word-ending *itis* implies that some sort of infection is at fault. It isn't that, as a rule. It is what we know as "degenerative disease," or just plain wear and tear. And little if anything at all can be done to reverse or halt this kind of trouble, except to take some of the load off the joints. Lose weight, that is.

Obese people are poorer surgical risks. They do not react as well as they should to anesthesia because they tend to be shallow breathers—the result of "invisible fat" that crowds the air passages of throat and lungs. This, by the way, is why many heavy people have guttural speaking voices, and why they snore more readily than thin people—which isn't to say that some thin people can't do a window-shaking job of snoring.

And there are other problems. The liver, so important to the utilization of our food, becomes infiltrated with fat, loses some of its efficiency, is subject to disease. Diabetes is another hazard, an immense one. Eighty percent of diabetics are people who have been too fat too long. (Fortunately and significantly, in milder cases weight reduction alone is often all that is needed to keep the condition under control, and as long as weight is maintained at the proper level, many patients require no medication, either insulin or pill-type.)

In pregnancy, stillbirths are twice as frequent among obese mothers. Toxemia and hemorrhage after delivery is greater among fat mothers. Can there be any question of the importance of correct weight as a rule of health and long life? None at all.

I dare say it is a good thing that appearance, and the fit of our clothes, is such a common reason for reducing. At least it leads people to be concerned over excess weight. But the wise person will remember that proper weight is one of the cornerstones of health.

But how do we accomplish it? There's a wide gap between wanting to reduce and achieving it, as some millions of people will agree. The accomplishment is so difficult—or seems to be—that the public grasps hopefully at every new "diet" that comes along.

The constant appearance of "new" reducing gimmicks is, indeed, pretty substantial evidence of how unsatisfactory they all are. This year's enthusiasm blots out last year's disappointment. We can be pretty sure that next year's enthusiasm will come along to take advantage that this year's wasn't what we expected it to be.

Why is this? Because we all are such inveterate daydreamers. We want an easy way of doing quickly something that should not be done quickly. In this endless search for a panacea we blind ourselves to the simple but sure way of getting results.

Hunting for some special diet is *not* the way to reduce. All it does is keep us blind to the truth. It keeps us hopefully trying one thing after another that won't work or will work only temporarily.

Specifically, I do not believe that the overweight person should go on any sort of a diet until he has done something else first: Learned how to eat an amount that will maintain his weight without further gain.

That is the one thing that the proponents and peddlers of "reducing diets" or "plans" or "systems" never mention, yet it is the most important factor of all. Nothing will take its place.

Sellers of proprietary reducing plans like to promise, in one way or another, that you can "eat all you want and reduce," or that "calories don't matter," or you "don't need to count calories."

The implication is that there is a way to lose weight without reducing the amount you eat. This is baloney, any way you slice, boil or garnish it. The only way anybody gets fat is by eating more food than his body can use; trying to make up theories to the contrary is just as silly as it sounds. Fat has to come from somewhere. It comes from excess food.

If you are fat, you have been eating more than you have been using up, and you can be quite certain that you have a firmly established habit of eating more than you need. If you go on a "diet" or "crash diet," you no doubt will lose some weight, but you can be just as sure that when you stop the diet, you will go back to your old way of eating and begin putting on weight again.

That, in a nutshell, is the reason why it is fundamentally important, first of all, to learn not to put on weight. Once you have learned that, it begins to make sense to reduce, because then, after a period of reducing, you can return to normal eating without regaining what you have lost.

Ideally, it would be best to lose weight as gradually as we put it on. Practically, this isn't easy. Most of us find it preferable to concentrate on losing for some limited time, then "resting" and subsequently losing some more. This works if you never forget the importance of not sliding back up in weight during the resting periods. Alternately losing and gaining it all back is not only a waste of time (and a waste of letting out or taking in waistlines of your clothes) but is also a pointless strain on the body and health. For another thing, this sort of up-and-down weight-changing means periodic stretching of the skin, and this in turn leads to flabbiness.

So take off weight, but be sure to keep it off.

Now how does a hearty eater go about changing his eating patterns? If he eats wisely, he can avoid the painfully severe hunger that accompanies crash diets. Protein foods are the type that "stay with you," because they digest gradually. These same foods are important for another reason. They provide the nourishment needed for strong, sound bodies, while other foods, starches and sugars, to be precise about it, furnish heat to keep the body warm and energy to keep us moving but provide relatively little toward building. Keep in mind that even at the age of 100 we continue to build our bodies, or perhaps I should say rebuild them, day by day, hour by hour and minute by minute. The very cells in our blood, for example, live only about 3 months, then are discarded and replaced by new ones. The same process goes on constantly as we replace our flesh, a microscopic cell at a time.

For these reasons a reducing menu should not skimp on protein —lean meat, fowl, fish and other sea foods, eggs, cheese and other dairy products. Bread contains some protein, but it contains a good deal more carbohydrate (starch). Of course, the eater who can put away two sirloin steaks at a sitting will do well to limit himself to one. It will be enough for his needs if not for his over-developed appetite.

However, those of us who have gotten along on an ordinary meat portion must look elsewhere for the cause of our excess weight. We can and should keep on eating normal meat (or other protein) servings but cut back on other things. And here come the carbohydrates—starches and sugars. Try limiting yourself to no more than one slice of bread or toast per meal. Incidentally, the food value of bread doesn't change by toasting it. A lot of "diets" make a point of including "dry toast." Bread would serve as well, except, perhaps, that the extra effort of chewing toast may give you a feeling of having had more to eat. (I doubt it.)

Put sweets off limits, except for the simplest of desserts. Cake, slice for slice, is far more fattening than bread because it is loaded with sugar. Apple pie is many times as fattening as an apple because of the sugar in the filling and the carbohydrate and shortening in the crust. The only safe rule is to quit sweets entirely, except for something on the order of a gelatin dessert, or plain fruit.

This alone is enough to correct a good many eating habits to the extent that no other change need be made. It won't work, though, if you let a sweet tooth tempt you into breaking the rule. You can't skip desserts and make up for it by eating candy. The rule has to be followed 24 hours a day, not just at the dinner table.

This might be a good place to remind ourselves of the three distinct types of overeating. Some folks, poor souls, overeat in all three ways.

First, one may simply eat too much of everything.

Second, he may not eat an excessive volume of food, but he eats only high-calorie foods: starches, sugars, fats (highest in calories, ounce for ounce, of any foods), cream soups instead of consommé, lots of butter on bread, potatoes and vegetables, cream in the coffee, whole milk instead of skim milk.

Third, one may eat proper amounts of the correct foods at mealtime but spoil the whole program by nibbling between meals. The handful of crackers, the candy bar, the sandwich, the leftovers from the refrigerator—these add up to the difference between enough food and too much.

How do *you* eat? Which of the three ways should you change? That's the first step in changing your eating pattern. Once you thoroughly understand it, the matter of weight control becomes a great deal easier than you had ever supposed. Too often people realize that they ought to reduce, but they don't do it because they have in their minds the idea that losing weight means an agony of being hungry. It needn't.

While discussing the pesky between-meals snacks, I'll mention two other common dangers. One is the practice of nibbling, more common among women but not limited to that sex. Around the house, it is the easiest thing in the world to nibble and to do it so automatically that you don't realize you are doing it.

You clean out the odds and ends in the icebox, and you don't like to waste the half portion of this or that. You eat it. Cutting up bread to stuff the chicken, you nibble a crust. You taste what you are cooking. You lick a finger from the frosting bowl. None of this is a crime. But all of it means more calories.

This is the explanation for some few very-hard-to-reduce people who swear by all that is holy that they are sticking to their 1,000 or 1,200 calories a day and who still get fatter. They think they are sticking to their calorie limits, but they honestly don't realize that by tens and twenties and fifties they are adding some hundreds of calories a day. But the body has its own adding machine that never makes a mistake in keeping track of what actually reaches our stomachs.

In treating weight problems some doctors have even gone so far as to put such people in the hospital, under strict supervision, to prove to them that they really have been eating much more than they thought they were. It's an expensive way to do it, but it works.

Now for the second kind of "nibbling," or should we say nipping? It's surprising how many people forget to count liquids as food. They casually toss off a hundred calories in a glass (or sometimes more, depending on what is in the glass) without the slightest realization that they might as well have been dipping into the candy box. Pop, ginger ale, lemonade, cola drinks and all the rest of them are sweet. They are sweet because they have sugar in them. (More recently low-calorie beverages of this type have become available).

Beer is a high-calorie drink. Straight liquor, ounce for ounce, is much higher. Many a "business man's bulge" wouldn't be there at all if only he would eat exactly as he did 25 years ago and would omit all his martinis at lunch, his highball or two when he got home from work, his drinks at the evening bridge table, his nightcaps before going to bed, his beer and his hot dogs at ball games. You have to be just as smart as your metabolism. Your body knows a calorie when it meets one. If you don't count all the calories, whether liquid or solid, that you swallow, your arithmetic won't come out even with the inveterately accurate addition of your body chemistry.

Thus our rule for normal weight changes again slightly. It now reads like this: Cut down your daily intake until it is just enough to balance what you use. Then, at times, reduce it still more so you actually lose weight. Then return to your steady-weight eating. Later on you can lose some more. But don't, *don't* let yourself be fooled into trying to deceive that unfoolable adding machine in your stomach. Don't think you are fooling anybody by thinking up goofy arguments to allow yourself an extra martini, an extra cup of coffee (with cream and/or sugar) or a glass of ginger ale or cola, without having it added onto your calories. You can't fool nature.

There's an allied classic bit of self-deception practiced by thousands, or maybe millions, of us. It's the trick of rationalization. We want an extra drink, or a sundae, or a piece of pie, or a teentsyweentsy box of candy, and we justify it by saying, "Yes, it's calories, but I'll just have juice and coffee for breakfast tomorrow." Or, "I won't eat any potato for dinner." This latter is especially attractive if it happens to be some kind of potato that we don't especially like.

Learn to school yourself in this sort of trickery. Learn to know when you are kidding yourself. Along with it, you probably will find some tricks which will work *for* you. It's old stuff, but still sound, to learn to reach for a stalk of celery or a few carrot sticks or a wedge of raw cabbage when you feel the urge to munch on something. One of my newspaper readers said she had solved that problem by sucking a piece of an ice cube at such times—no calories at all! It isn't, with a well-planned menu, true hunger that makes you want to eat. It is merely the desire to eat something, and there is a very real difference between hunger, appetite and the wish to eat something. If we ate only when we were really hungry, nobody would get fat. Or very few.

In the psychological realm there are all sorts of reasons for overeating. We eat because we are bored, lonely or frustrated. The child who eats to compensate for a lack of affection, whether real or imagined, is a familiar classic type. The same thing can affect adults, too, naturally. It is one form of "compulsive eating" (being driven to eating because of emotional drives). There are all sorts of variations, but they all come down to the same thing: satisfying one basic urge (the urge to eat) to make up for lack of fulfilling another urge, or masking despondency, worry, anxiety, continued tension, frustration.

There is another form of compulsive eating which deserves mention for the sake of completeness, even though it is rare. Injury or infection which affects the midbrain, where the appetite center is located, can cause compulsive eating. It takes skilled medical diagnosis to identify this situation.

Glandular upsets are possible but are blamed far oftener than the truth warrants. Once in a great while the excessively fat (and usually sexually underdeveloped) child is the victim of faulty glandular development. Under skilled medical observation this can be determined accurately and corrected. But it is rare, and it is self-delusion to use it as an excuse for letting a child, or anyone else, remain fat. Indeed, when, as too often happens, someone uses the excuse in conversation with me, my reaction is this answer: "If your trouble is glandular, why do you put up with it? Why don't you have it treated and corrected?" Glandular trouble is not an adequate excuse, you see.

All the same, as I have mentioned before, I regard it as obvious that we do not all utilize food in the same fashion. Within rather narrow limits, some of us absorb more and some absorb less of the nutritive elements as they pass through the digestive system. This again is an appealing but deceptive excuse for the person who is trying to rationalize his refusal to reduce. For if a person truly absorbs food more fully, he doesn't need as much food. Elementary, isn't it—as well as alimentary if you'll pardon the pun?

Thus 95 percent, and perhaps more, of the cases of overweight can be attributed to the bare fact that we eat more than we need or should, and the only answer is to learn to eat less.

I've distributed many thousands of leaflets outlining more briefly than in this book the inescapable importance of learning to know how much we can eat without overeating. From time to time I receive very pleasant letters telling me that the idea, when sincerely used, works. I have also, once or twice, received irate letters from readers who have said, "I think you are a fake," or words to that effect, "because what you say is that the way to reduce is to eat less. Well, I already knew that!"

If they knew it, why didn't they abide by the facts? The answer is that some people, even when they know better, still believe in pixies, perpetual motion, get-rich-quick schemes, something-for-nothing offers—and ways to lose weight while still eating like pigs. For them, nothing can be done.

But I want to add one more point about this matter of learning how much you can eat without eating too much. For a variety of reasons, this cannot be done by "counting calories." True, the caloric content is of vital importance, but how are you going to keep track of it mathematically without a complicated bookkeeping system, and carrying scales to weigh every bite? You can't.

Neither can you calculate, with such arithmetical precision, the amount that *you* should eat, without taking into consideration your size, the amount of exercise you get and so on. Use calorie charts as a guide, so that you automatically recognize the high-calorie and low-calorie foods. The common-sense way, at that point, is to be a scale-watcher. If your weight continues to rise, you are eating too much. By this form of checking, you soon learn to gauge automatically your correct food intake.

A word of warning on scale-watching. Weigh yourself at the same time of day. Women often take on a little added weight (occasionally quite a lot) in the form of fluids accumulating in the tissues just before the menstrual period. This is lost afterward. So don't be misled by this periodic and temporary fluctuation.

In that regard, menopause receives wholesale blame for weight gain. A sample letter:

> I am 42. At 24 I had a hysterectomy. It is hard to keep my weight down. The thing that bothers me most is the shape of my abdomen. What could be done to have a flat tummy?
>
> *L.T.*
> Maryland

I chose that letter from among thousands because it illustrates a much-misunderstood point. The hysterectomy at age 24 constituted what we call "surgical menopause." The removal of the ovaries accomplished surgically what Mother Nature does naturally at menopause. But the overweight problem did not accompany this surgical menopause. Instead, it developed at 40 or thereabouts.

It isn't the menopause that adds the weight. It is age and the things that go with middle age. We slow down. We don't burn up energy by staying up late for parties, by working our heads off to get a start in life and establish a home. Our children are grown. We have acquired household devices to save work. We like to sit and read or watch TV instead of going bowling, swimming or hiking. But we keep on eating at the rate we always did. Sometimes we eat more and richer foods because we don't have to count the pennies as we did when we were first married.

We learn how to "make our heads save our heels." And unless we alter our eating habits to conform, we put on weight. It may not be much. Say, the difference is only an ounce a day. In a year this is about 15 pounds. In two years, 30. Thus in a period of several years, only a fraction of an ounce a day is the difference between a good figure and an oversized one. Keep that in mind while you watch the bathroom scale. And keep it in mind when you hear a fat person say, "Why, I don't eat any more than Mary does, but she doesn't have her food turn to fat the way mine does." Enough exercise to burn up half an ounce of fat a day from the body, or the wisdom to avoid the snacks that add half an ounce a day can be the difference. Such factors as these usually *are* the difference. Understanding this can give you the assurance to realize that staying at normal weight does *not* involve starvation or hunger.

But if you must shed 10, 20, 30 or more pounds, you have to accept the fact that you are undoing what has been done over quite a few preceding years.

As to exercise, B.C. of New York wrote: "I am 35 and overweight and trying to reduce. Would like to know if exercise every day would help me reduce or is reducing strictly a matter of diet?"

The answer is that certainly exercise helps, but if you expect exercise to do it all, it will mean several hours a day of hard, vigorous work. For all practical purposes, the sensible way is to combine both exercise and reduced food intake. Elaborate studies of overweight people showed just what we might logically expect. The heavier people become, the less they move around. Conversely, the less weight they have to carry, the more they tend to move about. It all adds up.

This also is the answer to the letter from L. T. whose concern was how to have a flat tummy. First of all, fat has favorite places in which to accumulate, and the abdomen is one of them. There is some variation from person to person in the natural shape of the body, and some difference, but not a great deal, in the distribution of fat. By and large we react pretty much the same way.

To make a bulgy tummy flat, lose some weight! And exercise those abdominal muscles, because, as the fat departs, exercise is the only thing that will tighten up the stretched, flabby muscles and tissues. Neither exercise alone nor dieting alone will do it all for you.

What kind of exercises? It doesn't really matter very much, if you make those muscles work. The simple trunk-bending exercises that many of us learned in school (bending forward, back and sidewise) are excellent.

A favorite is to lie flat on your back on the floor. Raise each leg or raise both legs together, keeping them straight. Hold the legs up for 10 or 15 seconds at a time. Then repeat. This will tighten abdominal muscles and is good for the hips as well. A variation is to lie on your back and move your legs as though riding a bicycle. Push-ups, bending and touching your toes and similar exercises are all good. The important thing is to make those muscles work—hard!

Finally, what about "special diets," pills, gadgets? The "seven-day diets," "Hollywood diets" and "special food" notions sound easy, but they are usually futile unless you know the pitfalls and can avoid them. The same is true of fasting—temporary starvation is what that amounts to.

I am frequently asked, "What do you think of my trying the egg diet—eat nothing but eggs for a week or 10 days? I have a neighbor who says it is wonderful. She does it regularly, once or twice a year." Sometimes it's bananas, grapes, or another food, instead of eggs. Yet it all comes to the same principle. If you have to go on one of these radical diets "once or twice a year," something is wrong. You lose weight by starvation or semistarvation. Then you go back to your old eating habits. And you start gaining again.

The only truly valuable "reducing system" is one that teaches you to train your appetite—to acquire the habit either of eating less or of eating foods of lower caloric value.

Look up the word *diet* in the dictionary. You will find that it is defined as *mode of living* or some such phrase.

I think most people will be far happier if they never use crash diets but regularly cut down enough to lose a single pound in a week or so, then eat normally, then take off another pound. It's better for the disposition as well as the body, and it avoids the risk of following a diet so restricted that it lacks sufficient protein, vitamins and minerals.

The Council on Food and Nutrition of the American Medical Association has made a searching study of many devices and "systems" offered for reducing. Some involve exercise, which is fine. But be suspicious of promises about what massage will do. You can't rub fat off. Further, "spot reduction," or removing fat only from hips, thighs, chin, neck, and so on, while leaving the rest of the body the way it is, is not possible. Exercise can make loose muscles taut. Practicing good posture is most useful. But you can't pick and choose the places where fat can be magically made to disappear. It will come off in much the same order in which it went on.

Baths involving steaming or baking the body can cause temporary weight reduction to the extent that profuse sweating rids the body of water. Water is heavy. Several pounds can be "lost" at a time. It promptly returns. It will return even if you try very hard to drink no more fluids than you usually do. Why? Because your body, made abnormally short of water, will tend to hang onto what little it gets until the former balance is restored.

Don't skip meals. First, it disrupts the correct and adequate routine of eating which you hope to acquire. Second, it makes you crabby, disturbs normal, healthy digestion and elimination. Third, it results in your eating more at the next meal, making it still harder for you to accustom yourself to eating just enough, neither too much nor too little.

Some "systems" involve eating a piece of candy before a meal, the theory being that it will take the edge off your appetite. I doubt if this has any effect other than the psychological effect of calling your attention to the fact that you then *must* eat less dinner.

Finally, there are "pills." As a generality, these medications suppress appetite and increase activity. They vary in strength, but are of the amphetamine group of drugs. Used to excess—and some people are more sensitive to them than others—they can be dangerous. Sleeplessness, nervous jitters and irritability are among the more frequent side effects.

I cannot protest the use of these medications if they are used under medical supervision to avoid harming the patient's health. That must be a matter of choice. However, it is my observation that most physicians resort to the use of such drugs only at the insistence of patients who expect wonderful and "easy" results, or in cases in which patients simply will not exert the thought and will power to accomplish the required results in safer and surer ways.

The real reason for avoiding these pills is of a somewhat simpler nature. What, you must ask yourself, are you going to do when you stop taking the pills? It is certainly impractical to keep on taking them indefinitely. Once the pills stop, have you learned anything about the correct way of eating? No, you haven't. You go right back to the eating habits that cause trouble in the first place.

So thus again we come back to the same fundamental rule. No matter how you lose weight, learning how much food will keep your weight steady is the one thing you cannot omit without failing.

There isn't any other way. There is no pot of gold at the end of the rainbow except one. The "pot of gold" in reducing is learning to accept the basic truth.

After that, but only after that, does weight control become successful and, in a matter of months, easy. Once that single precept is thoroughly mastered it is just as easy to keep your weight steady at 120 or 140 pounds as it used to be to starve yourself intermittently to stay below 175 or 200.

Easier, in fact. Much easier.

4

LET YOUR HEART BEAT

MAXIM 4 *Know how to take care of your heart.*

Centuries ago the theologians used to spend endless time arguing the question of "How many angels can stand on the point of a pin?"

You get into just the same pointless and unanswerable argument if you try to reason out whether the heart is the "most important organ in the body." Or to put it another way, it's like arguing whether the front wheels or the back wheels of a car are more necessary.

However, of this we can be sure: When the heart stops, life stops. And of all causes of recorded mortality, heart disease and disease of the blood vessels are the two most frequent, leaving cancer in third place. If we are smart about caring for our health, we will take the trouble to understand how the heart operates, what diseases damage it, and what we can do to prevent (or correct) such damage. Diagnosing and treating heart trouble can be a task of great difficulty in practice. Understanding the fundamentals, however, is quite simple.

The heart itself is, essentially, a large sac of strong, muscular tissue. In an adult it is slightly larger than a clenched fist. It is

55

not, however, a single sac. It is divided into four chambers, each with suitable valves.

When the muscle of which the heart mainly consists contracts, a heartbeat or systole occurs. The contraction forces blood out of the chambers. Because of the valves, the blood can flow in only one direction, forward. The muscle then relaxes (diastole).

Blood collects in the first chamber, is forced from the second chamber into the lungs to be refreshed by oxygen, returns to the third chamber, then passes into the fourth and final one. From there it is forced out into the arteries to make a new circuit of the body.

In a lifetime the heart pumps millions of quarts of blood, working day and night. Because a brief pause is included in each cycle of its pumping action, it actually rests one-third of the time. Nevertheless, it seems amazing that a heart can go on working for 75 or 100 years without faltering. From another standpoint, it is not so remarkable. Nature wisely fashioned the human body to withstand the stresses that it must meet. The muscle which makes up the important wall portion of the heart is immensely strong.

Indeed, it has been calculated that the young and healthy heart is something like thirty times as strong as it needs to be. Thus it has a tremendous reserve of strength to meet sudden demands, to withstand the ravages of disease or injury and to keep on beating for perhaps a century in spite of the wear and tear of the years. *If protected from damage* the heart can easily go on beating much longer than the Biblical three score and ten years.

To be practical about things, what are the kinds of damage that can occur? And how can we protect against them?

THE HEART MUSCLE ITSELF

The durable heart muscle is, obviously, a basic element of the heart. Although it is built with an immense reserve of strength, that does not mean that its reserves can never be exhausted. They can. It isn't hard work that "wears out the heart," but some flaw in the organ or in its blood supply.

Like every muscle, the heart (or coronary) muscle must be nourished by a blood supply. If something shuts off that blood supply, the muscle is soon damaged, for the heart muscle, unlike so many other muscles in the body, cannot stop and rest when it is damaged or deprived. It has to go on beating, getting its rest in the periods between beats.

The heart muscle, because of its importance, is equipped with its own blood supply flowing through what we call the coronary artery. The coronary artery branches off from the aorta (the main artery leading from the heart itself).

Now don't become confused by visualizing this coronary artery as a single, long tube. It isn't. Rather, it resembles the pattern of a tree: a main trunk, dividing into large branches which in turn divide into smaller and smaller branches down to twigs and leaves.

Shut off this main artery, and death occurs within minutes. However, this rarely happens. Instead, the circulation may be shut off (by an embolus or clot lodging in the artery) at some point farther along in the "tree." Only a portion of the muscle is affected. The rest of the heart muscle continues to receive its normal blood supply and keeps on beating.

That part of the heart muscle from which blood has been shut off, however, becomes infarcted—another way of saying that the muscle tissue actually dies and is gradually transformed into a hard, scar-like type of tissue.

This is what happens in the "heart attack" we hear so much about. It is also called a "coronary attack," or "coronary occlusion," meaning that the coronary artery at some point has become extremely narrowed or obstructed. Or, in common parlance, we often speak of such an attack as simply "a coronary."

The "coronary infarct" or "coronary infarction" refers to the resultant damage to the muscle.

If the heart withstands the shock of the original occlusion, it gradually begins to regain strength.

The area of infarct, to be sure, never recovers. But the rest of the heart muscle does. Keep in mind the immense reserve power in the heart.

That is why 75 percent of persons who have had coronary attacks ultimately go back to their regular jobs. Immediately after the attack they usually are kept in bed, as inactive as possible, to put the least possible strain on the heart while it is recovering.

Some areas, marginal so far as the damage goes, may have been deprived of some but not all of their blood supply. These areas can show some recovery, if blood supply can be restored—and that is precisely what logical Nature attempts to do. All of our flesh is honeycombed with extremely small blood vessels. This is true of the heart muscle, too. These tiny blood vessels, some almost microscopically small, gradually enlarge and presently carry a helpful amount of the blood supply, which had been curtailed.

That is the story of a heart attack, and that is why you may have known people who were struck down by heart attacks, barely clung to life for a time, then began gaining strength again.

Naturally, when a series of heart attacks occurs, the damage becomes greater with each one. Hence, such precautions as we know about are advisable after a heart attack as well as before.

How to Avoid Heart Attacks

Preventing heart attacks depends, quite obviously, on knowing what causes them. I must admit frankly that we do not know as much about the causes as we wish we did. However, better that we use what we do know than waste time regretting what we don't.

Basically, a narrowing and/or hardening of the blood vessels is the underlying cause of a heart attack or, for that matter, the clogging of a vessel anywhere else in the body.

As we grow older we all experience some degree of atherosclerosis. This is a little different from the thing we used to hear a good deal about, arteriosclerosis, or "hardening of the arteries."

Atherosclerosis, rather than being simply a hardening or brittleness of the arteries, includes also a thickening of the inner lining of the arteries. Fatty material accumulates in the form of plaques or patches on the inside of the arteries. The same sort of material can also accumulate *in* the artery walls rather than only *on* them.

The arteries do, in fact, become "hardened," in that they lose the pliability of youth, but, in addition, the plaques actually reduce the size of the arterial opening, just as lime deposited in water pipes makes the space through which water must flow smaller. The plaques do not appear uniformly but build up more rapidly in some places than in others. The point at which an artery branches is such a place. The build-up can cause extreme narrowing, down to the diameter of a pin. The artery may be narrowed by unusual stress (activity) of the heart muscle. The amount of blood getting through becomes inadequate for the muscle area supplied. Then you have trouble. This condition may occur gradually, giving warning symptoms or changes in the electrocardiogram, or may appear suddenly.

How can we prevent it? There is no pill, no quick treatment, no vaccination against this sort of thing.

It has been facetiously remarked that one good way of avoiding a heart attack is to make sure that you have parents and grandparents who had excellent arteries. This is a factor, a significant one. But since we can't change our ancestry, our next best move is to be increasingly careful and to start being so increasingly early in life, if we know that our ancestors were prone to such troubles. Our arteries, after all, don't become caked with these fatty plaques all of a sudden. It is a slow process, continuing year after year. What takes a long time to happen usually can't be undone either quickly or easily. It is so here.

The way to protect your arteries and, therefore, your heart is to adopt some health rules early and stick to them.

First, keep your weight normal. Excess weight is the enemy of any heart that is having trouble. While it will be helpful to shed excess weight late in the game, it is immeasurably better to do it early in life.

Second, get regular exercise. Again, don't wait until you have signs of trouble. Stay in the habit of getting regular, if not necessarily heavy, exercise every day.

Third, there continues to be considerable question as to how much effect diet has. Excessive amounts of cholesterol and other fatty materials in the blood stream appear to play a part in the rate at which atherosclerosis develops. Whether diets, no matter how rigid, can reduce cholesterol and other blood fats to the degree that it will make any real difference, is the question. It is questionable whether a change in diet can reduce atherosclerosis, once it has occurred. Perhaps, at best, it can limit the rate at which it progresses.

On the other hand, a diet which is limited in cholesterol-producing foods will not be harmful. Therefore my feeling (subject to conforming with whatever further information may be developed) is to eat carefully but not to go overboard.

The long-range pull is the important thing. A violently restricted diet, followed for only a short time, means almost nothing.

The rule of thumb for knowing which are low and which are high cholesterol-producing foods is quite simple.

The high cholesterol-producing foods are animal fats. Those low in cholesterol production are, in general, fish or vegetable fats.

Another handy rule is to remember that fats which are solid at room temperature tend to be high in saturated fats. Those that are liquid at room temperature are low in saturated and high in poly-unsaturated fats. The saturated fats are the chief building blocks for cholesterol.

The rule is not absolute. Some margarines are being made with poly-unsaturated fats, yet the consistency is about the same as butter, which contains butterfat—a saturated, animal fat.

Eggs, it is true, contain cholesterol, but I am strongly inclined to worry very little about eggs. Why? Because the yolks (the cholesterol portion) are pretty well balanced by other materials (lipotropic agents) which put cholesterol into solution and transport it through the system more readily. For another reason, it is not my opinion that very many people overeat where eggs are concerned. An egg or two for breakfast isn't out of line. Furthermore, the human body needs a reasonable amount of protein under any circumstances, and eggs are a good source of it.

Thus diet-wise, it is my feeling that a person has done all that is likely to be of value to him in that regard if from his twenties on, he has kept his weight normal and has been habitually careful not to eat too much animal fat. A reasonable rule is: If your weight was normal at age 30, this is a good weight for the rest of your life.

THE VALVES OF THE HEART

Now let's move to another aspect of heart disease, the valves. We've already discussed their purpose—to keep the blood flowing in the same direction.

There are all sorts of technicalities, but essentially there are two kinds of flaws in the valves: Either the valve won't open sufficiently, thus retarding the flow of blood and making the heart work too hard; or it won't close tightly, and with each beat some blood is forced backward. This means that the same blood has to be pumped twice.

The greatest single cause of damaged heart valves is infection, and rheumatic fever (a form of streptococcus infection) is at the top of the list. It has been most gratifying in the last several years to see real attention being paid to rheumatic fever, and effective treatment being given as soon as the disease is identified.

Not every sore throat is rheumatic fever—but it is mighty rare to find rheumatic fever without discovering that it has been accompanied or usually preceded by a "strep sore throat."

A particular form of the streptococcus germ has the savage habit of going far beyond the throat. It causes arthritic pains in the joints, brings about changes in the blood and inflames sensitive areas of the heart, especially the valves.

The damage takes place not only in the initial attack but also during the aftermath. As the inflamed areas heal, leaving scars, the scar tissue itself can make the valves stick or can alter their shape so that they no longer close tightly.

Subsequent attacks of the same disease pile damage on damage, and one attack of rheumatic fever is fair warning that another will occur if the patient again encounters the same bacterium.

The answer is to start giving a long-lasting type of penicillin after the first attack. It is now possible to inject one dose a month; protection against the strep will remain from one injection to the next. I know of no other sure method of conquering rheumatic fever, but it must be started before permanent heart damage has occurred. After that, all it can do is prevent more. It cannot undo what has been done. If the individual is sensitive to penicillin, other mycin-type drugs may be used.

With this, I have offered about all that the patient can do for himself in the way of protecting the heart valves. From there on he must depend on his doctor or his surgeon.

In recent years, particularly since the maturing of open-heart surgery (during which a mechanical heart permits the surgeon to work with the heart in full view while the pump maintains circulation), surgical repair of damaged valves has been making great progress. It is even possible, in some cases, to substitute plastic valves when the real valves have been damaged too much.

In other instances, plastic surgery is employed to reconstruct a faulty valve. In relatively simpler cases, although no heart surgery can be truly described as "simple," a "frozen" valve may merely be forced open, after which it moves with sufficient ease.

I see no point in going into the great intricacies of such surgery here, but I do want to point out that the dangers of faulty valves are at the least twofold. Obviously a leaky valve will force the heart to do much more work than it is supposed to do.

But another danger is this: With the valves not working in balanced harmony, distorted pressures develop—too high here, too low there. Since the blood is pumped through the lungs, if pressure backs up into that area, the lungs can become permanently damaged from being forced to work under such conditions.

There are cases, therefore, in which correction of such valves may be urgent, even though the patient may feel that he is "getting along all right" and wants to put off the operation. You might wait too long—so if you are told of such reasons for hastening surgery, keep in mind that they are valid. It is not a case of someone trying to hurry you into having an operation.

CONGENITAL HEART DEFECTS

Now let's talk about congenital heart defects, the kind with which some babies are born. Some of them are valve defects. Sometimes the blood vessels, for unaccountable reasons, connect to the heart in the wrong places. Sometimes the sinuses or dividing walls between adjacent chambers of the heart have imperfections, ranging from small to quite large leaks.

There are several variations of these faults or flaws, and surgeons are still discovering ways of correcting some of them. Some defects, such as the "interventricular septal defect" (a gap in the tissue between the two lower chambers, or ventricles) are commonly encountered in modern operating rooms.

Some more easily corrected defects, which cause the so-called "blue babies," were being diagnosed and corrected surgically in Baltimore before World War II. Some extreme defects remain hopeless—so far. But doctors are struggling constantly to find ways of correcting the more difficult errors of nature, and every few months or perhaps every year or so now, we hear of some startlingly adroit method of curing some child who hitherto had been in the class of, "We're sorry, but we can't yet treat this type."

There are at least a few thoughts I want to impart to parents of children needing heart surgery. There is, naturally, a risk involved in the operation. There is at least a trace of real risk in the simplest surgery, even in having a tooth pulled.

When a baby is blue in fingers and lips and is gasping for breath, too weak to play the way an ordinary child does, it is not as difficult for the parents to accept the risk of surgery as it is when the child shows little or no outward sign of heart trouble except, perhaps, being unduly tired by exertion.

Obviously, (although there are distinct exceptions) the latter cases are, in general, more ticklish to handle than the latter. Since a child may seem to be in reasonably good health, parents often delay surgery, advised (or sometimes misadvised by all the aunts, uncles and neighbors within hearing) to wait in hopes that "the doctors could be wrong" and the child will grow strong and healthy without surgery.

The diagnosticians these days can predict with mournful precision the youngsters who, to their parents, are only "frail," yet are doomed to be invalids or dead by the time they are in their teens or twenties.

X rays, electrocardiograms, the stethoscope, respiration measurements and that wonderful technique, heart catheterization, permit very exact definition of the condition of a heart defect. As the years pass we are finding that forecasts of what will happen, with or without surgery, are being borne out.

The catheterization test, which terrifies some parents but doesn't upset others at all, is, really, one of the extremely useful ones. A vein in the arm is opened, and a thin rubber tube (the catheter) is gently slid through the vein until it reaches the point at which returning blood enters the heart itself.

So does the catheter. It is possible to get samples of blood for analysis, and possible to measure the pressure at very exact points inside the heart. It provides information obtainable in no other way. While the idea of inserting a tube into a child's heart (or an adult's!) is the sort of thing that can give some of us the jitters, the risk is actually slight; the information so obtained is beyond price. If the child were mine, I would say "Yes" without hesitation to a heart diagnostician who suggested catheterization.

THAT "TERRIBLE HEART PAIN"

Now let's move on to one of the most distressing types of heart pain, angina pectoris.

This is a chest pain—indescribable to one who has not experienced it but unmistakable to a patient familiar with it—that usually starts in the region of the heart and may even extend through the shoulder and down the arm.

It is, by and large, a protest of a coronary muscle that is deprived of adequate blood flow. I do not mean that it is a sign of a coronary attack. Likewise, the patient may or may not have had a coronary in the past. Usually he has had some sort of heart damage.

The heart muscle is getting enough sustenance (that is, blood circulation) to maintain it if the heart does not have to do very much work. But force the heart to work beyond the adequacy of the blood flow, and it rebels with this painful spasm of the muscle.

In the interests of accuracy, I must add that angina pectoris sometimes occurs in patients in whom we can find no diagnostic trace of heart disease. This is something we still do not understand, but it happens.

Incidentally, this may be as good a time as any to emphasize that the human body is not a machine. It does not lend itself to the absolute sort of analysis to which an electric motor, a TV set or a gasoline engine responds. A machine doesn't have nerves. It isn't dependent on the interplay of hormones, blood chemistry and enzymes. It doesn't have emotions playing strange tricks. You can take a machine apart, look inside and test the constituents one at a time.

It has been said again and again, yet perhaps not really understood by the general public, that medicine is "a science and an art." It is not solely either. It is a strange wedding of the two, with sometimes one, and sometimes the other, dominant in a given case.

A doctor, possessed of all the factual information about a particular patient, still has to know some of that patient's quirks and peculiarities, some of his habits of exaggerating or minimizing his symptoms, something about the way the individual's fears and tensions, or lack of them, behave.

Even then, it may still be necessary to modify a particular treatment if it doesn't help the patient adequately. This is part of the fascination, not to say frustration, of trying to treat the ills that afflict humanity.

With some kinds of things, as the congenital heart defects that we discussed earlier, it is possible to find that blood flows in certain amounts and certain pressures in specific channels, and it is possible to predict with great assurance what the result of the defects will be in the future. We may not be able to say that the end result will appear in any given year, but we can foretell it within a span of several years.

Angina pectoris can be another sort of problem, because it is a matter of spasm and cramping pain and is not subject to being measured the way we can measure your temperature or your heart rate, the amperage in an electric cable or the horsepower of an engine.

However, we can say in most cases it is a matter of lack of adequate circulation, with a few cases presenting something of a mystery. Spasm of the arteries, which slows down circulation to some degree (yet does so without any physical heart damage being present), is one conceivable explanation for some of these cases.

But let us take the average case. The patient is subjected to exhausting sieges of pain, particularly when he overdoes a little. "Overdoing" for such a patient is not at all like "overdoing" for one with a normal heart. Eating a meal, walking a block, going up or down stairs can be enough exertion to push the heart past the load it can carry without rebelling. In some instances it may be several blocks of walking—in which case the important secret of comfort is to get the patient to know exactly how much he can do or how far he can go without exceeding his limit.

If he can learn to walk half his maximum distance slowly, then sit down and rest for a time, he can go the rest of the way. He must also learn to evaluate his own nervous tensions, because they use up energy. He must learn to remember that digesting a meal requires diversion of circulation to the digestive tract, and he must figure on that.

There are also more severe angina cases, with the patients waking from a sound sleep to feel an attack starting.

For any of these, nitroglycerin is a very useful medicine. A tiny pill placed under the tongue gives the laboring heart a temporary boost. The smart patient learns to know when he has just about reached his limit, so he can take a tablet just before the pain is about to start and thus stall it off.

Certain nitrite compounds also are used for the same purpose. There are some differences in the speed and duration of help from them, therefore your doctor may try you on more than one form of medication before deciding which is best for you. But the purpose is entirely the same.

One of the most frequent questions I receive from patients (and their close relatives) is whether these nitro or similar pills are "habit-forming" or harmful in any way.

The answer is an unqualified "No." They are not habit-forming. They are not narcotics and in no way are related to narcotics. They are not, in fact, a pain-suppressing medication in the usual sense. They stop the pain of an angina attack solely by giving the heart a brief boost so that it stops hurting in protest against being overburdened.

Neither do they lose their effect from repeated use. They can be taken as often as the pain indicates they are needed.

Unfortunately, they do not correct the underlying problem, which is insufficient circulation to the coronary muscle.

Attempts have been made surgically to transplant other arteries, or otherwise to direct more blood flow to the hungry muscle. Results have not been as conclusive as we might wish in many cases, but we do have on record patients who have been afforded substantial relief from such procedures. Work in this direction is continuing in a number of centers, in the hope of perfecting such operations.

For the present, however, nitroglycerin or similar drugs continue to be the most reliable treatment. Success with them depends to a very large extent upon how well the patient understands what brings on the pain and what the capsules can do to relieve it.

The patient absolutely must, in other words, learn precisely how much work his heart can do before it starts to rebel. He must learn to rest before he has reached the point at which the sudden pain attacks. Even a defective heart, properly understood and cared for, is capable of still giving years of service.

WHAT "HEART FAILURE" MEANS

"Heart failure" or a heart "being in failure" is terminology frequently used medically, but for some odd reason its true significance is comparatively little known to people.

How often have we heard someone use the expression, "I was so frightened that I almost died of heart failure." The implication is that heart failure means a sudden and complete stopping of the heart.

Medically this is not the meaning at all. *Failure* means that the heart is unable to keep on pumping the amount of blood required for full normal activity of the body. The answer is to give such medical assistance as is possible and, in addition, teach the patient how to conserve his heart power, and make the most use of the capabilities that remain.

Heart failure results from a tired, worn heart muscle.

Causes? Changes may have resulted from faulty valves of long standing. The ventricle (lower chamber) enlarges because of the backwash of blood through a defective mitral valve. Its muscular fibers become thin and weak. It lacks sufficient force in the beat to push the blood into the general circulation. Similar changes can occur from high blood pressure of long duration. Or extensive damage from a coronary heart attack may involve so much of the muscle as to leave the remainder unequal to the task.

The sluggish circulation causes shortness of breath, congestion in the lungs, dusky nails and lips, swelling of ankles. The heart's thrust, however, can be given a boost with the useful drug, digitalis. Congestion can be relieved by use of diuretic (water-releasing) drugs. With such assistance, a tired heart can go on for many years.

More and more you have been seeing articles about patients with "Stokes-Adams syndrome." This is a fault in the human mechanism that governs the rate of the heartbeat. The heart beats so slowly that it does not pump enough blood. The ailment is not new; successful treatment of it, however, is. A "pacemaker," or machine that applies a carefully timed electric impulse to the heart, is used to speed up the rate of beat. Miniature pacemakers now have been developed so that such a patient can walk around with a pacemaker fastened in place, keeping his heartbeat regular.

One should not become panicky when the words *heart trouble* or *heart disease* occur. The same is true of *heart failure*. True, nobody wants to have heart trouble, but you would be surprised at the number of people, including some of your own friends and acquaintances, who are living contented lives, working regularly at their jobs and enjoying themselves despite some degree of heart trouble.

I lay special emphasis on this because taking heart disease in stride—accepting it for what it is, refusing to let yourself become "all nerved up" with fear—is one of the basic rules of keeping such cases under control. Looking at it from the doctor's viewpoint, the patient who is constantly demanding medication "to quiet my nerves" and is in a continuing emotional turmoil may thereby be undoing much of the good that would otherwise be accomplished.

Remember that!

You will, of course, follow whatever instructions are laid down for you and take pains to use, strictly according to orders, such medications as may be prescribed—if any. There are many heart cases that require little or none.

Get adequate sleep. Keep your weight at the correct level. Know how much your heart can do, and be careful not to overload it. But at the same time get as much exercise as your doctor will allow, which usually will mean the amount you can tolerate without huffing and puffing and becoming short of breath, and certainly short of the amount that causes pain.

WHEN A HEART "SKIPS A BEAT"

Through my medical column, as well as in personal contact, I have received thousands of questions along this line: "What does it mean, Doctor, when my heart skips a beat? Does that mean heart trouble?"

Or another question, "What can I do to keep my heart from racing? It comes without warning, but I feel as though it is just going to keep racing until I die."

Both of these, the racing or *tachycardia*, which simply means "rapid heartbeat," and the "skipped beat" are much more common than the patient usually supposes and, as a rule, very much less dangerous. Indeed, it is perfectly possible for either to happen without having any significance at all, healthwise.

The "skipped beat" ordinarily isn't really a skip at all. It is far more likely to be an extra beat. A "beat" impulse is transmitted ahead of time so the heart, after its regular rhythm, suddenly inserts a "beat-beat," or two beats close together, followed by a pause afterward. This is called an "extra systole," and the essential "treatment" consists of trying to find what may be causing it and of convincing the patient that it usually doesn't mean anything. For that is most often the case, and unless there are additional symptoms of some sort, there is no reason for alarm.

Tachycardia (a heart suddenly racing for no apparent reason) often falls in the same category: something that occurs by accident or because of nervous tension. There can be cases, it is true, when it signifies something more serious, but generally the first things to check are whether the patient is drinking too much tea, coffee or other drinks containing caffein, or smoking too much.

(When it comes to drinking "too much" tea or coffee, there is no fixed rule as to how much is enough. It varies from person to person. A couple of cups may upset one person, while another may have a cup or two several times a day without ill effect. Anyway, if rapid heartbeat occurs, try avoiding all caffein drinks for a few days and see whether the annoyance ceases.)

Still another cause, and one that can stand some correction, may be an overactive thyroid. This, too, is something that occurs more frequently than the average person realizes. Any wide discrepancy from normal in thyroid activity naturally demands skilled treatment. Lesser variations above and below may not warrant doing anything, unless they happen to cause some annoying symptom, such as a rapid heartbeat.

Another scary incident, for some people, is the sense of feeling the heart beat. Ordinarily we are so used to it that we pay no attention. But when we sit, or more likely lie, in a particular position, we may feel the thump-thump-thump of the heart, or of the pulse of blood as it surges through a major artery. Here again it usually means nothing. One of the few exceptions (an uncommon one) could be an aneurysm, which is a bulged-out place in the aorta. In such a case it is extremely probable that other symptoms would be present: perhaps difficulty in breathing, pain in abdomen or legs, trouble swallowing. Otherwise, forget it.

And let's dispose of one more question that keeps bobbing up: "Is it harmful to lie on your face or on your left side?" The answer is "No." The heart is contained entirely inside the rib cage. If the heart is not enlarged, there won't be enough weight to interfere with its action.

If the heart is greatly enlarged from disease, position may make a difference. The patient, however, readily senses this and learns which position is most comfortable.

Another common complaint about which I *cannot* be so reassuring is "acute indigestion."

There are so many of us who just don't know where the heart is. Ask someone to put his hand over his heart, and the hand is likely to land almost anywhere from floating ribs to the collar bone, and almost without exception too far to the left. The heart is *not* positioned behind your shirt pocket. It is underneath the breastbone and—like some French political parties—only just a little left of center! We are brought up from childhood to believe that heart pain is going to be located somewhere in the left part of the chest.

At the same time we associate pain arising in the heart with "stomach distress." That is why many a serious heart attack does not receive attention as soon as it should. The victim feels intense, cramping pain and ascribes it to indigestion. He'll take some fizzy antacid, perhaps, and rest awhile. Instead the pain continues and grows worse, and sometimes he collapses before anyone recognizes what probably ails him.

A few tips on the way a coronary attack develops, and what to do about it, ought by the law of averages to be helpful sooner or later to a good many readers of this book.

The pain is at first usually continuous but may not always be. The likeliest place is underneath the breastbone, but it may start at first in the shoulder or even in the arm. It may be in the shoulder-blade area only. It is also a little difficult to point exactly to the site of the pain. You know it approximately, yet when you try to show the exact point, you often realize that this is impossible. There is an intensely painful sense of pressure, relentless dull aching or constriction, accompanied, as a rule, by considerable shortness of breath, sweating and pallor of the skin.

There is very little that you, as a layman, can do except to summon a doctor and let him know the urgency. Let the patient lie down wherever it is easiest for him. Avoid every possible bit of physical exertion on his part. If he is cold, cover him. Don't try to give any medication or stimulants.

Since he probably will have difficulty breathing, loosen garments (tight collars, and so on) that may restrict respiration.

Beyond that, do nothing except to reassure the patient. It is quite common for the victim of heart attack to have a strong feeling of impending death. Death usually does not occur, although in a massive heart attack, it can come very quickly. The fact is that approximately 80 percent of those who have suffered heart attacks survive—and we have no way of knowing how many more survive lesser heart attacks without realizing at the time what is happening!

Keep the patient quiet and calm, tell him that the doctor is on the way and that he will soon be feeling better.

As a matter of fact, he won't be out of the woods. Any heart attack, even a relatively mild one, must be treated as potentially dangerous, yet several times as many survive as do not. The patient is in for an extended period of bed rest and observation.

But you will be telling him the exact truth when you say that he will soon be feeling better. If he is still in pain, as quite usually he will be, the doctor will give him some powerful sedative to ease the pain, let him relax and perhaps even nod off asleep.

By the time he becomes aware of what is going on around him again, he will be safely tucked in bed and starting his recovery. For the nature of such an attack is such that the first elements of recovery are starting about the time he has passed through the acute stage!

It is folly to speak of mild or light heart attacks. I think they are all serious at first. Certain symptoms give the doctor an indication of *how* serious an attack threatens to be. These are: the degree of shock, status of the blood pressure, failure to respond promptly to adequate treatment.

THE TOOLS OF CARDIOLOGY

Finally, let's have a word or two about the tools used by the doctor in ascertaining the condition of your heart. First is the familiar old stethoscope—still an essential instrument, as it has been ever since the French physician, Laennec, invented the first crude model in 1816.

All it provides is sound amplification—of the sounds in the chest, the faint gurgles and rushing noises as the valves open and close, and as the blood courses through the heart. It also gives, by means of the sounds of breathing, some indication of the condition of the lungs. It can, within rough limits, indicate where a sound originates.

But it can't do everything. X ray is the second great tool, for it can give very precise answers as to the size and shape of the heart. Enlargement of the heart indicates that there is, or at least has been, some abnormal strain on the heart—that the heart has become larger in its attempt to compensate. Enlargement of some chambers but not others can give excellent indication of where pressures have gone too high and perhaps can point to a means of restoring pressures to normal again.

Third of the valuable instruments is, of course, the electrocardiogram (ECG, also called EKG), which will disclose information that neither of the others can, although it cannot substitute for the others. Faint electric impulses are constantly running along the nerve and other muscle tissues of the heart. The wavy, rising and falling line on the ECG record is much more than a matter of the rise and fall of these tiny voltages. The pattern is significant. Irregularity of beat, of course, will show. So will other abnormalities. The aftermath of a coronary attack, for example, will be clearly visible to a physician trained to read this wavy line. Indeed, many a coronary, unsuspected at the time, is discovered afterward by means of the ECG.

My point in all of this is to make clear that no single instrument can tell the whole story. Irregularities detected by stethoscope and ECG may, for example, indicate the need for X rays to disclose more specific data. When you "pass" a physical examination with these instruments you can be reasonably certain that your heart is in good working order.

The one big item that sometimes (but by no means usually) escapes even such a searching examination is the possibility of the dangerous coronary. Why can't we always see it coming? Probably for more than one reason. With our present knowledge, we usually can tell with at least moderate accuracy when the arteries are becoming unduly laden with the plaques of atherosclerosis, but we cannot foretell when a major obstruction will develop any more than we can predict, say, being struck by lightning.

Another difficulty in this type of prediction may well be—probably is—the fact that motion in one or another part of the heart is almost perpetual. The human body isn't a finite thing like the plumbing system in a building. It is dynamic. There can be momentary pressures here or there. This may, in some cases, cause a momentary narrowing of an artery at some point yet not necessarily reveal itself in a single X ray or series of X rays or electrocardiograms. Given the right or, to be exact, wrong set of circumstances at the exactly wrong split second, it is no doubt possible for damage to take place—damage that would not have occurred at some other moment in time.

Can we someday hope to detect such subtleties as these? Yes, there is hope in that direction. Within the last decade or so, high-speed X-ray equipment has been developed that can take a series of pictures at intervals of a split second.

At the time of this writing, cardiologists are now making headway with still another method: the combined use of fluoroscope and a camera to make a continuous recording, just as television programs can be recorded or taped and then run at will. Equipment known as an "image intensifier" is also utilized in this process, so that only a very small amount of radiation is required to bring out a good, clear picture.

In at least one research center, pictures are taken simultaneously, from front to back and from side to side, so that what amounts to a true three-dimensional representation of the heart is then available.

The tapes can be filed indefinitely, permitting comparison of the conditions of a heart at various intervals. It should, and I feel certain will, be of immense value in greater understanding of exactly how the heart behaves or sometimes misbehaves.

But it may prove to have even further value. Since the whole cycle of the heart's action can be recorded and subsequently rerun for detailed re-examination at will, we may someday be able to detect in advance even those coronary attacks that today occasionally still strike without warning. Some research doctors of high repute have gone so far as to suggest that exactly this may come about.

This particular work is in its relative infancy, but I could not resist including it here as an example of the way in which medical science continues to press forward toward answers to problems that continue to plague us.

5

BREATHE FREE

MAXIM 5 *Don't let "lung failure" rob you of health. A few simple precautions will add years to your life.*

The time is surely coming when we will all be doing a great deal more to prolong the usefulness of our lungs, and that means prolonging our lives. The pity is that today millions of people are not aware of the precautions they can take *now* to add years to their lives, and to add even more years to their *useful* lives.

How many people are aware of such things as emphysema, bronchiectasis and hyperventilation? How many understand that asthma, unless controlled, is a threat to the heart itself? People who are now battling such problems know that there is a great deal more to "lung disease" than we used to think, back in the days when the very term was taken as synonymous with consumption or tuberculosis.

Letters to me via my newspaper column are beginning—and it is high time—to include more questions like this:

Dear Doctor:

I have just learned that I have emphysema. I hope that is spelled correctly. I never heard of it before, but it is making me very short of breath. What can I do about it? Is it curable? What causes it?

R.J.T.

Yes, emphysema is spelled right (and pronounced em-fizz-zee-ma). And of course it make him short of breath; that is the fundamental symptom of this disease. Nor is R.J.T. the first or the last person to admit that he never heard of it before. Everyone is going to hear a great deal about this problem in the future. It is already so prevalent that some authorities are saying that it kills more victims than tuberculosis and lung cancer combined.

Emphysema is a loss of elasticity in the lungs. To understand why this is a peril to health and even to life, we'd best review the physiology of breathing.

When we take a breath, what we really do is exert force with the diaphragm, opening the lungs to greater capacity. It is just like drawing air into a bellows. Air rushes in.

We exhale simply by relaxing. The springy lung tissues contract to their original size, forcing stale air out.

What happens when the lungs lose their ability to contract? They do not force the stale air out. Instead, like a balloon that has been blown up too often and has lost its stretch, the lungs simply hang slackly, still containing much of the air that had been drawn in.

By the laws of physics, two things can't occupy the same space at the same time. If air is already in the lungs, fresh air can't be drawn in.

To be sure, the patient with emphysema manages to expel some air and to draw in an equivalent amount, but he does not get nearly as much fresh air as he should.

He struggles to get a full breath; over a period of time this constant effort gradually brings an actual expansion of the chest. The victim may appear to have "a big, or barrel, chest." Unless what really has happened is understood—that there is loss of ability to exhale—it can be difficult to comprehend that the victim is being starved for air. Starved for *fresh* air, that is, for his lungs remain full of air depleted of its oxygen content saturated with carbon dioxide instead.

How to Combat Air Starvation

The letter we're discussing asked, "Is it curable? What causes it?"

Emphysema may have a number of causes. Why one person develops it and another does not depends on their exposure to certain factors and the stamina of the lung tissue. Repeated infection or irritation of the bronchiole tubes, with intermittent coughing, is one cause. Heavy smoking may thus be a factor. Some physicians refuse to accept an emphysema patient for treatment unless he stops smoking completely. Exposure to irritating fumes or dusts can be another cause. Most patients with asthma have some degree of emphysema, as well. Glass blowers and musicians who play wind instruments have, in the past, been noted as somewhat more likely to develop emphysema.

There is no cure for emphysema. Rather, we try to relieve the distress and to prevent further damage to the lungs. Trying to put the "stretch" back into the lung tissues is as frustrating as trying to put the stretch back into a rubber band that has become brittle and has no snap. (I do not, however, imply that the lungs become brittle.)

As the trouble continues, the blood does not get enough oxygen as it passes through the lungs. In turn, the tissues of the entire body cry out their physiological signals, demanding more oxygen. The heart responds by working harder, but merely circulating oxygen-poor blood at a faster rate avails little. The lack is not blood; it is oxygen. In time, obviously, the heart must begin to fail under this unrelenting burden.

Does this seem like a gloomy outlook? Well, it is. This is a dangerous disease, and we aren't going to do any good by hiding our heads in the sand. We must face the fact that first comes shortness of breath, huffing and puffing over what should be minor exertion. More severely afflicted patients become invalids, or semi-invalids, unable to work. Finally, the disease can cause death, and it is doing so more often than is realized by people who have not yet had occasion to know about emphysema.

For all this, there are things we can do about it, even if we can't cure it. We can't cure diabetes or pernicious anemia or a good many other things, either, but we can do much to control them. (In the two diseases I just cited, both of which once were extremely deadly, patients now, with proper medication, live out their normal life spans; often even close friends do not realize that any illness is present.)

We cannot yet undertake to do that well with emphysema. On the other hand, emphysema rarely affects young people. The patient very likely has little or no suspicion of what is happening until he is in his forties, fifties or sixties, for we are born with considerably greater lung capacity than we need.

A person who isn't especially athletic can lose as much as three-quarters of his "breathing ability" before he really begins to notice that anything is wrong. A rather simple test, however, will provide early warning that trouble is starting. The trouble begins, remember, with a decline in the ability to expel air from the lungs. What, then, would be more logical than to rig up a device that will measure the amount of breath expelled in a half second or second? That, indeed, is exactly what is being done with devices known as "spirometers" (several other names have been devised for such instruments). These machines are simple enough for the individual to use: he just takes a breath, then blows into a mouthpiece leading to a tank. Some lessening of an emphysema patient's ability to exhale will show on the readings long before he can begin to notice any deficiency himself.

Others who have had impairment of breathing creep up on them, frequently tell of having experienced some shortness of breath or a nagging cough for some time.

Treatment of emphysema should be started when the disease is in an early stage, not after it has become disabling. Fortunately, a variety of methods are available.

First, and most obvious, is to give up smoking. Whatever lung space is filled by smoke or fumes of burning tobacco is space subtracted from that available for fresh air.

Further, rocking beds can be used to help breathing while the patient is lying down or sleeping. These beds have been used for

other types of breathing difficulty, including cases in which polio
has partially, but not entirely, paralyzed muscles used for breathing. The so-called "positive pressure" devices for getting air into
and out of damaged lungs are put to good use.

Since the lacking element isn't really air but is its vital constitu-
ent, oxygen, great relief is also afforded by giving pure oxygen.
Some patients keep small tanks in their homes. I have known
others (some of whom were required to do considerable traveling
in their work) who carried small oxygen tanks with them from
city to city.

Patients with emphysema tend to breathe with their abdominal
muscles. Occasionally, the use of an abdominal binder forces
greater—and hence beneficial—use of the chest wall muscles for
breathing. In any case, the patient should make a conscientious
attempt to use his chest muscles more.

These measures, singly or in combination, can make an enormous difference. In some cases, brief treatments, perhaps 15
minutes or so, in the morning and evening are sufficient to give
enough "lift" to keep a person both comfortable and active
throughout the day.

If appropriate, drugs may be used to suppress infection that,
by causing swelling, may curtail the space in the air passages
through which the breath must flow. Some physicians prescribe
antibiotics periodically for short intervals. In addition, drugs to
dilate the bronchial tubes and to loosen thick secretions (making
coughing easier) are used.

In still other cases, showing the patient how to improve his
posture is an effective aid.

The net result not only is more comfort and activity for the
patient but also relief from the endless burden of trying to gasp
enough air into his lungs. Since we breathe something like 20,000
times a day, the struggle for breath adds up into a great deal of
sheer physical effort in 24 hours.

Finally, it goes without saying that increasing the total oxygen
intake by any or all of these methods is bound to take excess
burden off the laboring heart. We husband the body's total
strength instead of letting it be sapped.

FROM THE TIP OF THE NOSE

It may appear that I have devoted an inordinate amount of discussion to this single disease, emphysema. Perhaps I have, but not without reason.

For one, this is one of the lung diseases that only now is beginning to receive substantial attention—partly because there is every indication that it is increasing. For another, emphysema brings out a number of aspects that become very useful in discussing other respiratory ailments.

The respiratory system extends from the tips of our noses to the bottoms of our lungs. Consequences of lung disease are known to have a pronounced effect upon the heart; the indirect results, of course, have impact on the entire body.

We are, quite rightly, hearing a lot about "preventive medicine" today. The respiratory system is an ideal area in which we can all practice preventive medicine in ways that will count. However, I have a nagging suspicion that the majority of us have not really fixed in our minds what "preventive medicine" is.

It isn't all up to the doctor! He must, obviously, be given a chance, but he can't do it all himself. How do we go about that? The ready answer is, "Have a regular physician—and go to him for periodic checkups."

Sometimes puzzled readers have written to me saying, in one way another, "All my doctor does is take a few minutes to examine me, tell me to watch my diet and tell me I'm fine. What's so preventive about that?"

The answer, if these people would look a little deeper, isn't hard to see. True preventive medicine doesn't mean that you have to find something wrong every visit. Good health isn't a TV thriller that has to have a crisis in every installment.

Rather, it is a methodical, continuing search for the *first sign* of something going wrong. Let's face it: There's nothing healthy about a morbid suspicion that this, that or the other thing *might* be wrong with us. You doubtless know somebody who has that attitude. I know countless people like that. They are sure they have cancer, or "know the doctor didn't tell me the truth" or are "certain that the doctor didn't find what is really the matter with my stomach."

To my way of thinking, that must be a miserable way to live— and certainly not a sound way to guard your health.

The healthiest, happiest people I know *expect* to be healthy most of the time. There is no question that tension, worry and "nerves" have their effect on our physical health—in ways, I grant, that are subtle and not too well understood, but we know it is so.

Expecting to have normally good health, taking the few but basic steps of eating, sleeping and exercising correctly, and having a periodic checkup to catch any intruding symptoms early is the way to enjoy vigorous good health.

Your doctor need not go into a great deal of elaborate and costly testing if you and he, together, have achieved a sort of team attitude—which should exist between every patient and his physician.

At this point I freely concede that big industries now quite universally have their executives go through exhaustive checkups once a year. This gained its impetus first during World War II, when disablement of a key executive could wreak havoc with a vital defense program.

Subsequently, it has become apparent that this is good business, well worth the money. A couple of days a year devoted to the closest medical scrutiny is a small price to pay if, perchance, a month's illness can be avoided, or if an extra-early detection of a stomach ulcer can prevent a month or two of having an executive working at half speed instead of full speed.

Futhermore, from my own experience I would point out that issuing specific orders to arrange for a thorough examination is the only way to get some of our high-powered industrial managers to have an adequate examination at all. Too many, I'm afraid, otherwise become so wrapped up in their jobs that they "can't afford to take the time" unless they are forced to.

But for the other 99½ percent of us, our regular physician can do a pretty effective job (and save the patient money while doing it) during a periodic checkup. The physician can see a great deal more in a small space of time than the patient suspects. Skin texture, color of the nails, the sound of your breathing, your posture —all tell their part of the story at a glance.

Unexplained loss of weight, a slight fever that hangs on and on, a murmur in the stethoscope or a raspy sound in your lungs— these and other swiftly absorbed facts point to the need of further examination. Or their absence lets us dismiss possibilities of danger.

Blood pressure readings, the simple urinalysis and blood count, for women the "Pap smear"—by the time you've been through these, your physician has a pretty dependable view of your general health.

WHAT TO TELL YOUR DOCTOR

Of decided importance also are the questions he asks you and the things you tell him. Let's take it for granted that your doctor already has your medical history on file: That in itself is a guide to which health areas need special attention.

Your doctor's questions are deliberately chosen to cover a lot of ground in a short time. Don't hold back any facts! If he asks, "Are you sleeping well?" he doesn't want a description of your having been awakened last week by somebody banging garbage cans around in the alley at 3 a.m. But he *does* expect you to tell him if you have a pattern of waking up drenched with sweat, or of having to get up repeatedly night after night to go to the bathroom, or of waking with a feeling of being unable to catch your breath.

If there is some unusual point that you have noticed, even though it doesn't come up in his questioning, tell him. Not trivialities, of course. But pain anywhere, excessive coughing, sore throat, a sign of blood anywhere, any continuing change in any of your bodily functions, unusual fatigue—anything, in short, that you really notice.

In the natural course of events, most of these will have little or no significance so far as any important health aspect is concerned. We all have aches and pains. But when a pain continues or is repeatedly present in a certain area, it becomes important. Pain is one of the things that protects us.

One more thing. Make use of community facilities which are designed to detect symptoms that need investigation. There are Diabetes Week programs and certain others that provide tests at no cost.

The most important of all brings us right back to respiratory conditions.

For years health departments and tuberculosis societies have been sponsoring chest X rays. They have helped make a tremendous dent in the ravages of this disease. In less than a generation we have seen the death rate from TB whittled down by 90 percent —although the number of cases has not subsided as rapidly as it should.

The societies can fit the X-ray machines into trucks, and park at factory gates, schools, in front of the city hall or on a main downtown street. But they can't make people spend the five minutes it takes to go in and have an X ray taken.

Do so! It saves you money. It may save you from tuberculosis. It may even save you from some other affliction quite unrelated to TB. If some unusual condition is noted, that fact will be passed along to your doctor. Heart abnormalities, for example, sometimes are detected. (In this regard, a word of warning: Some enlargement of the heart, or an abnormality in shape may be reported when, with subsequent examination, it is found not to be dangerous. That original X ray isn't the complete answer to anything. It isn't a diagnosis. It is only a tool for screening out such conditions as may require further study, so don't become panicky just because you receive word that you ought to see your doctor. It can be nothing.)

Recently, however, the TB societies have been changing their goals, their methods and even their names. They are calling themselves "Tuberculosis and Health," or "Tuberculosis and Respiratory Disease Societies."

It means no diminution of watchfulness for tuberculosis. Even though the death rate has come tumbling down, as long as we continue to find 100,000 new cases a year in the United States, we aren't being careful enough. We need more, not fewer, people walking into the doors of those X-ray trucks.

However, the trucks are doing much more than looking for

TB. More and more are being outfitted with respirometers or vitalometers, the breathing devices that I discussed in relation to emphysema earlier in this chapter.

The X ray usually provides suggestive clues to the presence of emphysema. The measurement of the amount of breath you inhale and exhale will give an additional index of trouble. Whether it is emphysema or something else depends on further diagnosis.

A study in Philadelphia showed that five times as many heavy cigaret smokers as nonsmokers had measurable inability to inhale and exhale a normal breath. The figures, incidentally, were 6 percent for nonsmokers, 15 percent for those who had given up smoking, 20 percent for cigaret smokers, and 12 percent for cigar and pipe smokers—with the figure markedly higher for those who were heavy cigaret smokers, meaning a pack or more of cigarets a day.

After years of smoking, I have quit because, in view of such figures as these, it seemed sheer foolishness not to. I won't argue the point, though. I'll just leave it with you.

I will, however, repeat my other point. Make use of X-ray and testing facilities. This service began as an attempt to battle what was a very deadly disease, tuberculosis. However, TB has lost much, but not all, of its deadliness; therefore, the campaign is now extending to other diseases or varying degrees of morbidity and mortality.

Without possible question, the breathing-test devices are going to be of immense value in improving the health and activeness of a great many people, quite in addition to saving numbers of actual lives.

ASTHMA—A PROBLEM OF ITS OWN

From babyhood to extreme old age, asthma can be a problem; it is more serious than some folks appear to realize.

The time to stop it is at the earliest possible age. Yes, sometimes it is outgrown by a child, and when I learn of such a case, I heave a sigh of relief and make a mental note that the doctor and parents undoubtedly have been wise in their handling of the situation. It isn't often easy.

Perhaps the greatest stumbling block to correct care of asthma cases is a misunderstanding of what it means. Specifically, it is a narrowing, due to spasm, of the branches of the bronchi (breathing passages) or "bronchial tubes" and the still smaller divisions or bronchioles.

To give you an example of exactly how *not* to regard this condition, take this letter drawn at random from questions on this topic:

Dear Doctor:

My son, 8 years old, has asthma so bad. It comes and goes. Several times I have had him to the doctor but it only helped for a little while, and then the attacks come back again. What medicine can I get that will keep his throat from closing up? It is so sad to see him trying to get his breath when one of these attacks is on. I have tried several remedies from the drug store but they don't help, either.

Asthma is not an infection, not a sore throat, or a variety of a cold. Rather, the bronchial tissues are hypersensitive to something, and they become swollen and congested as a result.

In other words, it is an allergic sort of thing. We have different responses to allergy. We may break out in a rash, our lips may swell, our noses run or tears flow. We may itch, sneeze or get hives. Congestion and obstruction of the bronchi may occur in some of us, causing wheezing and struggling for breath.

Cough syrups and "cold remedies" don't do a particle of good, any more than they would alleviate an attack of hay fever. To do any permanent good for a case of asthma, we have to take the longer view and find out what causes these attacks.

The most common offenders are things we eat or breathe—dust, certain odors, pollen, animal danders, for example.

It is heartbreaking to see a child having a severe asthma attack fight his frantic best to get enough breath to keep alive. There is precious little we can do for him, at the moment, except to comfort him, keep from becoming too frightened and sometimes give him an antihistamine compound of some sort to suppress temporarily the allergic reaction. Choice of such a medication is something that I certainly leave to your physician, since he will have firsthand knowledge of the case.

Keep firmly in mind that this temporary relief gives no protection against subsequent attacks and, indeed, does nothing to cure the basic trouble. It is a stopgap only.

The long-range improvement depends on learning what triggers these attacks, and either keeping the child from coming in contact with them, or helping him to develop sufficient tolerance to them. There may, and perhaps usually will, be a variety of things. Acute or chronic upper respiratory infections are common triggering factors.

True, children sometimes outgrow the attacks. Basically this means that they gradually become able to tolerate at least reasonable amounts of the substances or foods and can come in moderate contact without having an allergic reaction.

The finer points of this process are too complicated to go into here and are technical matters that, in any case, must be dealt with by your physician. For practical purposes relating to what we ourselves can do, fix this in your mind: As the child develops such tolerance as he is able to acquire, he should not be set back by being exposed to repeated onslaughts from the offending substances. In plainer English, if you discover that the child is allergic to eggs, wool or anything else, and your doctor wants him to be kept away from them, by all means do it. Tolerance, from an allergic standpoint, may build up. But every time there is a new exposure strong enough to bring on attack, it tears down some of that hard-won tolerance.

Then come questions like:

Dear Dr. Molner:

We live in _____. Would it be better if we moved to _____ to get relief from constant asthma attacks?

People in New England wonder about going to New Mexico or Arizona. Southern Californians wonder if the Midwest would be better. Midwesterners wonder if it would be better along the seacoast.

This climate question is a merry-go-round. Possibly one case in a hundred or one in a thousand—for all I can prove—might be benefited. There might, in some few cases, be something in the air in one place and not in another, so that a different part of the country (not strictly climate) might possibly be better.

The probabilities are so slim, however, that for practical purposes they reach the vanishing point. It is rare that a child is allergic to only one thing. (The same point applies to adults, too, of course.) If, for example, an asthma victim is allergic to something from palm trees, there is too much chance that a change in residence would prove only that he is also sensitive to something in pine trees, wheat fields or salt marshes. Better stay where you are unless an allergist can, with confidence, urge a change. Don't trade one trouble for another.

Still another aspect of asthma (and although this is not easily explained or comprehended, the evidence of its reality is overwhelming) is this condition's tremendously close connection with the emotions. Why this should be, I do not know. It applies to some forms of allergic disturbance and not much to others. Experts who have studied the matter most closely lay great emphasis on this emotional aspect. A person (particularly a youngster) who is subject to asthma attacks is likely to avoid them when things go smoothly from the emotional viewpoint but to fall victim to them suddenly when some nervous upset encroaches.

Don't ask me why; I don't know. But please note that I have mentioned earlier that our emotions have mighty effects on our physical reactions, even if we don't understand the reasons. This is not just a childhood reaction, either. For one notable example, observant skin specialists have long been aware that if they could calm the nerves of their patients, they often could curb their rashes, itches and other annoyances of the skin.

I think it's time somebody pointed this out, other than in medical meetings, where it is hardly new. Don't think your doctor is being fancy or far-fetched if he seems to spend as much time (or more) investigating the emotional reactions of an asthma patient as he spends on the purely physical manifestations. Such a specialist knows what he is doing!

On the more optimistic side of the coin, you should know that if a youngster goes into his teens with the asthma problem conquered, he has accomplished something important, and many a child does so. The armed forces, for one example, have their own "age deadline." They are perfectly willing to accept a boy who has had such trouble and overcome it. They are hardheadedly suspicious of the one who, as he enters his teens, still is seriously bothered. By that age, a pattern has been established, and while this does not mean that the battle cannot be won, it is harder and longer.

There are other facets to asthma. One in particular is cardiac asthma, an aspect of heart trouble. A heart which is not quite up to doing its required work is plagued by the fact that it cannot clear the body's tissues of excess fluids that normally should be discharged. In combination with other technical aspects that I will not elaborate, this can result in the accumulation of fluid in and around the lung tissues. Among other things, this can create lung congestion, or in some cases an "asthma," obstructing the little fingers of air space in the lungs. That is, after all, the definition of asthma.

Curtailment of oxygen in turn puts a greater strain on the already overburdened heart. A vicious circle? Of course it is! But that is the consequence of failure in a vital quarter. The heart bothers the lungs; the lungs return the compliment. It is the interplay of organs that is important, and I hope these paragraphs may save some long explanations by other physicians as to why a heart patient may be told that, unless he stops smoking, he is causing some of his own troubles.

PROTECTING NOSE AND THROAT

Taking care of your nose and throat is essentially a matter of logic and good sense, except for such instances as may require medical intervention.

Why do we have noses? One major service of the nose is to filter (as well as warm) the air we breathe. Millions of tiny cilia, or microscopic hair-like structures, line the mucous membranes, trapping harmful particles that then are gradually carried away by the mucus and cilia, instead of going into the lungs.

It makes sense, therefore, to keep our nasal passages in working condition. How? There really isn't much we need do except to pay attention when Nature needs help. The sign is obvious enough. We start breathing through the mouth!

In a child it may be adenoids or some structural defect. The deviated septum is one—the septum, or partition between the nostrils, is bent or forced out of normal position, interfering with the air passages on either one side or both.

There was a time when I, like others, had some reservations about surgery on the nose. That was years ago. Since then so much has been learned about such surgery that I do not hesitate to suggest it, because it is now so uniformly successful.

As we age, we find another problem that is more frequent than generally realized: polyps. These are soft growths, often described as "grape-like" (the growth emerges from the mucous membrane on a sort of stem). They may simply interfere with breathing, or they may be so located that they prevent proper drainage from the sinuses, that collection of cavern-like apertures that can ache so vociferously at times. Polyps in the nose are particularly prevalent in allergic individuals, so accept this as an important clue.

Removal of polyps, happily, is a matter of clipping the slim stem, ordinarily an office procedure not requiring hospitalization.

Sinus trouble, by the way, is not the mysterious ailment it is so often considered to be. The cavities are so placed as to suggest that Nature expected us to spend a good deal of our time on all fours, since in that position the openings are downward and drainage is easy. Cows, for example, don't have sinus trouble.

But we stand on our hind legs, with the sinus openings aimed more forward than downward, so that even a small interference is enough to clog the small apertures and cause pressure to build up inside. That is why parts of the face, eyes and forehead can be so painful.

Where polyps are the obstruction, removal brings rapid relief. In other cases, congestion is the result of some infection. Antibiotics, by suppressing the infection, relieve the congestion and pent-up pressure inside the sinuses. In some instances, physicians may use a hollow needle to drain a sinus, easing the pressure while the inflammation is being subdued.

Except for drugs to ease pain, medications are not likely to be of much use with sinus trouble, other than as temporary aids. The wise course is to find out precisely what is making it difficult for the sinuses to drain, and then to correct it.

A serious word of warning on this. Don't try to diagnose it yourself. It's hard to calculate how much misery comes of this, but it is a great deal. "Sinus" has developed into a handy catch-word, and there is a flourishing tendency for people to identify every headache and every attack of nasal catarrh as "sinus trouble."

Excessive smoking and nasal obstructions are two of the commonest causes of troubles glibly attributed to "sinus." Neither, naturally, will yield to any of the patent medicines or home remedies which so many people try. Nor will such remedies do much, if any, good with genuine sinus disease, either. Avoid self-diagnosis, and you'll find relief much sooner.

I must say much the same thing about the host of remedies for colds and flu. If I knew of a genuinely effective cold cure, I would certainly share the news—from the housetops. There are, to be sure, nose drops and pill-form medications which will dry up the nasal passages temporarily. As emergency drip-stoppers for some particular occasion, I can imagine using them—but sparingly. They do nothing to influence the course of the cold itself, and excessive drying of the membranes leaves them vulnerable to secondary infections—the invasion of random germs other than the cold viruses.

Since colds (as well as flu) are caused by viruses and not by bacteria, the antibiotics (antibacterial) drugs are of no effect. Because of this, the once overworked "shot of penicillin for a cold" has pretty well disappeared, I am happy to note. It was a waste of penicillin; it contributed to the risk of people becoming sensitive to that excellent drug; it may have done some harm in the sense that there was increased opportunity for some strains of bacteria to become penicillin-resistant. The only benefit, if any, was in suppressing secondary infections, and since most of us throw off colds in due time without any great amount of bacterial infection occurring, even this benefit was of limited value.

I hope we can look forward, in the coming years, to the development of cold vaccines, but (at this writing) such as exist are merely incidental to flu vaccines.

By now there should be no question about using flu vaccines for high-priority individuals: the old and infirm, those with chronic illnesses, pregnant women, people whose work is essential to the community. The younger people in vigorous health pull through flu pretty well as a rule, but an epidemic takes a high toll of lives among those in troubled health. Those who have chronic lung diseases, for example, certainly should take no chances but should have flu vaccinations every year at least.

For that matter, there certainly would be no objection to having everyone so vaccinated, for the vaccine probably wards off lighter attacks that could pass as colds.

Perhaps the fact to keep in mind is that there are scores of different viruses causing flu, colds, "grippe" and the like. Some sweep through in waves, like flu epidemics. Some pop up regularly, every year. Some, possibly, may well be scattered in varying intensities, either all the time or any time.

By encountering the diseases, we acquire temporary protection that gradually fades. Our natural physical resistance also varies. There are so many shades of resistance that the study of colds has been extremely difficult. In one classic series of studies in England, it was found that one person might—some of the time— be able to give a cold to another by being in the same room, but no success was met in attempts to transmit a cold by, for example, using material washed from the handkerchief of a cold victim.

I mention this not to get into the intricacies of virus studies but to suggest that we evidently catch our colds on a person-to-person basis—that sneezed or breathed droplets of moisture are sufficient to carry the living viruses short distances.

In our homes, or in familiar groups, we probably become pretty well adjusted to each other's germs. But when a member of the group brings in some of a new variety, they can spread readily.

By the same token, advice to avoid crowds in epidemic times is sound. I would add to it the thought that if you are extra-tired, have been up late the night before or haven't been eating as wisely as you usually do, it would be wise to stay at home or at least, for a day or two, have as little contact with other people as possible. You may well save yourself from exposure to cold germs at a time when your resistance is lowest.

My recipe for a cold cure? About the same that any other doctor will give you: aspirin, plenty of fluids, and stay home and rest. My one addition is this: If your face aches and your nose is sore and inflamed, pressing against it a washcloth soaked in water as hot as you can stand brings welcome if temporary relief.

Where a cough is severe and painful, a chest rub often may ease the discomfort, but is has no effect on the head cold itself.

Whisky or brandy for a cold? My answer is that if that is to your taste, and if it makes you temporarily less aware of your misery, that's up to you. It has no therapeutic value.

And the same for all the dozens or scores of "cold remedies" that are constantly being proposed by our friends. If you get any pleasure out of fooling yourself, and pretending that some pet potion helps, that again is up to you.

But I have yet to find the slightest scrap of evidence that discounts the old maxim of the medical profession: Ignore a cold and it will hang on for a week. Treat it, and you'll be rid of it in seven days.

PROTECTING THE THROAT AND BELOW

If you are one of the people who like to gargle, go ahead. I won't spoil your fun. But I do not think, except when a medicated gargle is being used for some specific purpose, that there is much benefit. Putting antiseptic on a finger an hour before you cut it isn't going to prevent infection. Antiseptics have to be used at the time of exposure to germs to be effective. Gargling, therefore, may perhaps protect you for the few minutes that you gargle. It leaves no lasting protection for the rest of the day. However, frequent, *hot,* weak salt solution gargles at the first sign of sore throat not only are soothing but may nip the infection early.

The best thing you can do to protect your throat and the bronchial tree—that spreading, branching pattern of air passages that reach into the lungs proper—is to observe the ordinary rules of good health and to take the hint when Nature warns you that this area is being irritated.

Essentially, this means a cough.

One letter from a worried wife gave me a wry feeling:

> Dear Doctor:
>
> My husband has a terrible cough but he absolutely re-
> fuses to go to a doctor or have a chest X ray. There has
> been so much about lung cancer and I have been begging
> him to see the doctor, but he says it is just a cigaret cough.
> Is there anything I can do?

No, in such cases I can't think of much to suggest except that perhaps it is one instance in which nagging is justified. Or some-times there can be some sort of a bargain. If he wants you to go fishing with him, or play cards or whatever it is, it might be bar-gaining material. You'll do it—if he'll agree to make an appoint-ment with the doctor. If he conveniently "forgets," make the appointment for him, and the stubborn character will have a hard time backing out.

However, it is the strange blind spot in this letter (and, believe me, many others like it) which disturbs me, too. Let's assume that the cough is "just a cigaret cough," and not lung cancer. Any way I look at it, this is no excuse for not doing something about the cough. The cough means irritation. Irritation means that some-thing ought to be done.

It may take 20 years or more for smoking to inflict enough irritation to create a cough. Fortunately, after a couple of weeks of not-smoking signs of relief begin to show. And I suppose if I said any more about smoking I would be wasting my breath.

Except that I can't help reporting what one physician said about his own motivation. He was, by the way, a former president of the American Cancer Society, so it was taken for granted, when he gave up cigarets, that he was just taking part in that society's consistent campaign to reduce lung cancer by reducing smoking.

"No," he said. "At my age, and after the length of time I have been smoking, I may be pretty late to be worrying about that.

"I stopped smoking so I could sleep nights—so I wouldn't wake up coughing."

Waiting for a cough is not the way to protect against lung cancer. The best way, naturally, is to remove as much of the cause as early in life as we can, and I think I see some rays of hope when I encounter young people who have stopped smoking or refused to start. There aren't very many, perhaps, but more will follow suit as time goes on.

Second best is detecting such a cancer while it is new enough and small enough to be removed. Surgical removal of a lobe of a lung, or even an entire lung, is being done every day now and is no longer the drastic and risky adventure it used to be. Not, you understand, that such an operation is a trifle, but it is being performed now with dependable assurance of success.

It's interesting to note that the techniques for such operations were perfected in tuberculosis hospitals; now they are being adapted to still other needs.

Lung cancer is sneaky and silent. Detection is primarily by chest X ray. Clues are persistent cough, raising of blood, and/or pain in the chest. The "Pap smear" has occasionally been used on sputum. Bronchoscopic examination, providing a direct look and possibly a chance to obtain tissue for biopsy, is a commonly used detection technique.

To get back to cigaret cough—why not call it bronchitis, instead of trying to floss it up with some other name? Bronchitis isn't to be casually dismissed. Recurrent coughing and clearing of phlegm from the bronchi is nuisance enough, but the more urgent reason for controlling it is to avoid its complications.

Many emphysema victims have a history of bronchitis. Is it because the coughing in time takes the "stretch" out of the lungs? I don't know, but it has a suspicious ring to it. Obstruction of the airways is a common complication of bronchitis, varying from mild to—at the extreme—fatal intensity. Respiratory infections are more frequent among bronchitis sufferers, and this includes pneumonia.

Pneumonia, to be sure, no longer is the terribly deadly disease it used to be. Now that we have antibiotics of various types for differing kinds of pneumonia, the mortality has declined to a fraction of its former frequency. Moreover, the illness is far shorter. A week or so in the hospital, or even treatment at home, is often enough to see the patient on the road back to recovery. It used to be a battle that continued for weeks, with the most intensive sort of nursing care.

There is one fly in this happy ointment. There were so many deaths from pneumonia in the past that the remaining fraction is still large enough to give us pause. If you doubt it, just obtain the mortality figures from your local health department. Pneumonia is still a killer, especially of older people, and doubly so for older people with respiratory ailments.

That is why I so seriously plead in this chapter that all my readers fix in their minds the importance of treating their breathing systems with reason and kindness. Take care of your nose, throat and lungs early in life, and they will serve you well in later life. And vice versa.

One last trouble, which certainly must be included, in view of its prevalence and of the number of inquiries I receive concerning it, is bronchiectasis.

Bronchiectasis is the commonest cause of coughing up blood. It is often the cause of foul breath, which harried people futilely try to combat with mouthwashes, toothpastes and so on. It may occur in children as a congenital defect in lung tissue development. More often it is an acquired disorder.

The bronchi, being soft tissues, sometimes acquire "pockets" or expanded, pouch-like sacs. The reason for this is not always clear. These pockets accumulate phlegm. They are liable to become sites for localized infection. This in turn increases the phlegm, of course. The victim finds his "throat" (really the passages below the throat) clogged, and he coughs and struggles to clear these passages. There may be offensive breath because the chronic infection creates puddles of pus.

Bronchiectasis can become an incapacitating ailment. In severe cases with extensive infection—and especially those with recurrent bleeding—removal of the affected segment of the lung affords relief and may be lifesaving.

Obviously, bronchiectasis demands the most careful and conservative treatment. Care requirements may be utterly simple or quite complicated. The patient, for example, may get an enormous amount of relief once he realizes the usefulness of lying, at times, with his head a little lower than the rest of his body. This permits the annoying material from pockets to flow gradually downward and be expelled, rather than agonizingly coughed up.

The patient must—and here comes this old smoking matter again—avoid further and continued irritation of the already inflamed or irritated areas. He will, if he can, spend most of his time away from smoky, fume-laden atmosphere. Along with this, the doctor will exert his best judgment as to which expectorants (cough syrups) will be most helpful, and which antibiotics will control whatever infection is present.

The physician will, I am sure, point out to the patient that plenty of other people have had bronchiectasis and that, although there is no way of "curing" the pockets, there are ways (if you work at it sensibly) of taking the sting out of the trouble.

To borrow a phase from the politicians, "If you can't beat 'em, join 'em." To turn it into a phrase that will help vastly more people, let's put it this way about diseases, "If you can't cure 'em, control 'em." This is a most useful rule, I hope you will apply it to other chapters in this volume.

6

YOUR BLOOD,
THE STREAM OF LIFE

MAXIM 6 *Understand how your blood serves you. Know what you can do to preserve its qualities.*

Even today I still get letters such as this:

Dear Dr. Molner:

Please give me the name of a good tonic, something that will purify the blood.

Mrs. T.Y.

Of course many of my readers well understand the futility of such a question, but a lot still don't. Shopping around for a "tonic for the blood" really is about like saying, "What should I use to wash a cake of soap with?" Our blood serves a number of purposes, and one of them is "purifying" the whole body.

We burn up much of our food in the form of activity. Let us, for example, take the muscles of the arm. Let's say that we are chopping wood or hammering nails and using up a lot of energy. How does the "fuel" for this reach the arm muscles? Why, via the blood, which carries it there in the form of blood sugar. There are some "ashes" left over. How do you get rid of them? The blood again!

In addition, the cells which make up the body are constantly being replaced, a few at a time. One cell dies off, and another cell divides in two—both then grow to the normal size. Debris from the discarded cells has to be carted away. The blood does it.

As the blood circulates through the millions of tiny filters in the kidneys, the wastes are extracted, then expelled in urine. A similar filtering action takes place in the lungs, where the blood is constantly discharging carbon dioxide and acquiring fresh oxygen.

Because the blood is constantly being thus purified by lungs and kidneys (as well as by some lesser factors), it is quite meaningless to think of taking a medicine or "tonic to purify the blood." The night-and-day, lifelong process of purification is being thoroughly taken care of.

I presume that some of this purification idea may come from the old but vague idea of having a spring tonic every year—the sulfur and molasses or other concoctions forced down the unwilling throats of youngsters.

A few generations ago, without routine shipment of fresh fruits and vegetables from other climates or frozen food techniques, and with only the limited facilities of home canning, people went through the winter being short-changed in their diets on vitamins, C and D in particular. The "tonics" were a blundering effort to "do something" about the diet deficiencies that people sensed but did not understand. They had nothing to do with the blood, but apparently a lot of people thought they did.

Another ambiguous phrase is "thin blood." Some people, who believe that there is such a thing, are ready victims of purveyors of nostrums offered to the unwary. The reference is probably to those who are anemic.

We still hear people say, "I've been in the south and my blood is thin. That's why I feel the cold so much."

Blood doesn't become "thinner" or "thicker" because of the climate. True, someone accustomed to warm weather may require a little time to get used to the cold, but it isn't because anything has changed in his blood. Blood is blood, and so long as no disease factor is involved, it is essentially the same.

That, of course, is why blood transfusions are possible, and why they are so effective in time of need. Human blood has to be matched for the correct "blood type," but aside from that it is interchangeable.

In World War II nobody asked whether blood (or plasma) came from somebody living in Arizona or in northern Minnesota. It just doesn't make any difference. (In practice, most of the plasma was and is from "pooled" blood, a supply representing a mixture from a number of donors. The fact that it can thus be pooled is another indication that blood is basically the same.)

Blood, to be sure, is a highly complex fluid. It makes up about one-eleventh or one-twelfth of our body weight—approximately 6 quarts for a person weighing 150 pounds.

How to Remedy the Anemias

Using a term that keeps popping up, one reader sent this inquiry:

Dear Doctor:

My doctor tells me I have very low blood. He gave me some pills and told me to eat plenty of good meat but that was all. What can I do to get my strength back faster?

Mrs. I.B.

This expression, "low blood," evidently comes from people who have been told that they have a low blood count, that is, a deficiency in the number of red cells or in iron content. Anemia is the general term for it.

The red blood count is possibly the most common diagnostic blood test, because anemia is frequent. A droplet of diluted blood is placed on a microscope slide, and the cells within a designated area are counted. If their number is markedly lower than average, the patient is anemic. A "hemoglobin determination" is another term, referring to iron content. Hemoglobin is the red, iron-containing material which holds oxygen while it is being transported through the body.

You may have noticed that I refer to "the anemias"; there are several different kinds. They all come down to the same thing: The blood is not capable of carrying enough oxygen. Yet the causes are varied, and consequently, different types are treated in different ways. There may actually be too few red cells—or the cells may not contain enough iron for their oxygen-carrying purpose. Diet, injury, poisons, illnesses—all these may cause anemia. That is why a physician may pay considerable attention to matters which do not, at first thought, seem to you to have much to do with your anemia.

For example, acute and heavy loss of blood, as from a severed artery, depletes the number of red cells faster than the body can replace them. The patient, in fact, is suffering from a sudden and extreme case of anemia. This can produce shock and death, if not checked.

Little realized by many folks, slow but continued loss of blood also can bring on anemia. The victim may not even realize that he is bleeding. A gastric ulcer, for example, can bleed slowly and give no sign of redness (although there may be black color) in the stool. When this is persistent it can cause anemia. So can bleeding hemorrhoids or "piles." Or excessive menstrual bleeding. Clearly, the cure is to correct the bleeding, not to try to replace the loss and let the bleeding go on.

There can be "anemia of pregnancy," probably related to the drain on the blood-forming capabilities because, after all, the foetus, or forming baby, must have its share. This is one of several reasons why diet during pregnancy should be watched somewhat more carefully. "Just eating a lot" is no answer, because gaining excessive weight in pregnancy is dangerous. But a diet with adequate protein, iron and calcium is very important.

Poor diet can lead to "nutritional anemia," a lack of sufficient iron, protein and vitamins. This, of course, leads to all sorts of other ailments, too. The answer is easy: Restore a normal diet, helping things along in the beginning with vitamins and iron.

Still another anemia is due to lack of iron. There are enough red cells, but all are deficient in iron either because enough iron from food has not been available or because the system—for one reason or another—does not absorb it well. This is the kind of anemia which calls for additional iron in the form of tablets, other pill types or liquid. Iron medication is not always well tolerated and can cause stomach and bowel disturbances in some individuals. Varying the type of iron medication may avoid this. If the source of blood loss is stopped and the diet adjusted properly, it may no longer be necessary to continue iron-containing medicines.

Next we have pernicious anemia, which until three or four decades ago was a terrifying disease because the patient wasted away before our eyes and there was nothing we could do. It was about as deadly a disease as any known.

Then it was discovered that eating great amounts of liver (a pound or more a day) would halt the disease. Arduous study revealed that there invariably is an absence of some vital factor in the systems of those afflicted with this ailment.

In time, it was found that liver extract contained this factor. Later, the factor was narrowed down to Vitamin B-12, and today an injection of this vitamin every couple of weeks or so controls a disease that used to be a death sentence.

Poisons (such as lead, arsenic and carbon tetrachloride), infections and excessive destruction of red cells can also cause anemia. I mention this last group briefly, just as a warning that, in a few cases, rare ailments differing in some respects from the more ordinary anemias may occur. They, too, have their characteristic signs, but leave that to your doctor to worry about. I'm trying, in this book, to give my readers some over-all views of the kinds of troubles we should watch for; if one of the rarer variations happens to appear, your doctor will pin it down. He has been alerted by his training and practice to look for the common ailments first, but to be forever watching for others that don't quite fit the pattern and hence must be investigated further.

SOME OTHER BLOOD PROBLEMS

Quite a variety of other blood disorders exist, nearly all of them not very common and some of them really quite rare.

There is one, however, that can be guaranteed to bring a succession of questions all year 'round, but more particularly when school is in session.

Dear Doctor:

My grandson is a student at Georgia Tech and I have just learned that he has been stricken with infectious mononucleosis. He is only 22, but is married and they have a baby and we are extremely worried as we are told that there is no cure for this disease.

You can readily understand the alarm that is generated when people hear that phrase, "There is no cure." Or, to be more accurate, undoubtedly the original statement from the physician was, "There is no specific treatment," which is quite true.

Yet there is no real cause for alarm, because the mononucleosis patient recovers fully, even with minimal care.

Mononucleosis (pronounced moe-no-new-klee-*oh*-sis, called "mono" for short, also known as "glandular fever") is what we know as a "self-limiting disease." In that sense it is like a cold; there is no cure but the disease runs its course, and that's the end of it. The one thing to watch out for is the appearance of complications—some infection may get started while the patient is weakened by the "mono," and then you have a different problem to meet. But that, of course, can be true of most of the diseases with which we contend.

It is strictly a blood disease, marked by the creation, at the expense of some other types of cells, of too many of a certain type of cell, the lymphocyte. The patient is inordinately tired. Glands swell and are tender. There is fever. Headaches, chills, sweating, tenderness in abdominal region are all possible symptoms.

Perhaps the one who comes down with a fairly hard and sudden attack is better off. A dean at one of the large universities told me about a student who, after having established himself as a very good one, was almost kicked out of school. His work went to pot. He missed classes, didn't turn in assignments, just seemed to lose all sense of industry and responsibility. It could have been disastrous until the dean insisted that he see a doctor. The belated answer: mononucleosis. The rest of that semester was ruined, but the boy went home and got a good rest. He was back in school the next term and did as well as he ever had before.

Treatment consists of rest (in bed while the fever remains), antibiotics to suppress complicating infections, medications to ease such symptoms as may be painful. Since the disease is infectious, if not acutely so, some care is warranted in having the patient use only his own eating utensils, towels and so forth. They should be sterilized with boiling water.

And presently the disease subsides and the patient gets back to normal. He should, though, watch for any of the familiar symptoms, because relapses can occur, and then it's the same thing all over again.

For whatever reasons, "mono" is especially common among teen-agers and young adults—in other words, those of boarding school or college age. Physicians treating groups of such students have learned to be very much on the alert for "mono."

Perhaps because it has such an unwieldy name, the existence of mononucleosis doesn't seem to stick in people's minds, and although I have written about it repeatedly, the supply of new and frightened inquiries never seems to run low.

I'm going to speak less of some of the other types of blood disorders, in part because they aren't very common, in part because there is so little you can do about them except to follow your doctor's instructions.

Leukemia is a dread disease. It is an overproduction of white cells, whose number may soar to 50 times normal or higher. The cells, furthermore, are not properly formed. For this reason leukemia is called "cancer of the blood," because cancer amounts to an uncontrolled or runaway formation of tissue cells, with the cells, likewise, not being correctly formed.

Leukemia can be either acute or chronic. The acute cases are almost always found in children. By the use of some powerful drugs it is now possible to force the acute disease into temporary remission. Indeed, for a time the situation is such that the youngster appears completely normal in every respect, and even the most detailed diagnostic tests may not show any sign of the disease.

But by sad experience, physicians have learned that this is temporary. In time the disease returns in full force, and this time it resists efforts at renewed remissions. It means that instead of only a few months of painful life, a child may have as much as a year or two, or perhaps even several years, of life, but it remains one of the most heartbreaking of diseases.

X-ray treatment, along with certain drugs, is most effective in suppressing chronic leukemia in adults, often for years.

There are varying diseases involving the clotting of blood, the most famous being hemophilia, the "bleeding disease" which has affected, among others, members of the Spanish and Russian royal families. Although it affects only males, it is transmitted through the female side of the family—a good sample of the intricacies of genetics.

As a rule, hemophilia runs in families, but there are occasional instances of it cropping up where no family history can be found. Equally baffling, sometimes a person with this disease finds that the ailment has left him for a time. It may be a few weeks, sometimes years.

Plainly, since it is a matter of the blood not being able to clot and thus halt bleeding, the primary goal (until we can find out the basic cause) is to prevent wounds, even small ones.

A little nick that occurs while we are shaving may be stopped in a minute or two. Five minutes, a little more or less, is enough time for the blood to clot and shut off bleeding from any except quite serious wounds. The clotting mechanism operates so swiftly that, for example, even in a very serious bleeding wound we will see an ebb and flow of blood. A clot starts to form; then it is forced loose, and we see it break free—followed by a gush of unclotted blood.

For all practical purposes, the hemophiliac must take every precaution against even nicks and scratches, because he will keep bleeding for hours instead of minutes. He must also be on guard against damage to joints and internal injuries, since bleeding in those sites can be serious. He surely will be equipped by his doctor with special materials to stanch the bleeding of external cuts, in case a small one occurs.

What Blood Tests Show

We've already discussed the red blood cell count in connection with its essential problem, the anemias.

Just about everybody is also familiar with the blood test required for people seeking marriage licenses. This is to detect the presence of syphilis, since the germ produces changes that will be found in the bloodstream of the person who has that disease.

The importance of the amount of sugar in the blood is being increasingly understood. Too high an amount usually signifies diabetes—the patient cannot make use of the sugar.

If, at times, the amount is too low (the term for this is *hypoglycemia*) then the patient either is using up sugar at too fast a rate or is not getting enough.

Blood sugar, remember, represents the fuel element of our food, which is transformed into energy or into heat. Low blood sugar manifests inself by intervals of feeling faint or weak, or having sudden periods of heavy sweating, abruptly "feeling famished" and the like.

The rate at which we use up energy can be measured in several ways. The familiar "B.M.R." (basal metabolism reading) is one. Compare the body to a furnace. You can measure the amount of fuel used. You also can measure (with the right equipment) the amount of air needed to burn the fuel. Either gives a record of the amount of burning.

Medically, the "B.M.R." measures the amount of oxygen we use. This is often done to determine whether the thyroid gland is properly regulating our metabolism. Still another test is used: the "P.B.I.," or protein-bound iodine test, which gives more precise results. It measures a certain type of iodine in the blood. If the thyroid is not sufficiently active, the amount of iodine will be low.

More recently, a new family of blood tests has become very useful for measurement of certain enzyme activities. Increased amounts of enzymes may be found in acute coronary heart disease, liver disease and pancreatitis. The rise and fall of the enzyme level gives a clue to the extent of damage to such tissues as are involved. And there are other, even more complicated tests. They are "blood tests" that seek quite different types of information.

Not all transfusions are alike. Some cases require whole blood. A striking example is open-heart surgery, in which an artificial heart or pump is used to maintain circulation while the heart itself is being repaired. Since there must be enough additional blood to fill the pump and connecting tubes, plus enough to make up for whatever is normally lost during the operation, plus of course some reserve in case of emergency, such operations require a large amount.

Except for such cases, however, it is not usual for patients to require more than perhaps 4 pints, and often less. There have been a few extraordinary instances in which, over a period of a few days, as many as 30 or more pints have been used, but such cases as these represented dire emergencies in which the patient was bleeding heavily and there was no quick way to stop it.

Other transfusions, instead of using whole blood, use plasma—the fluid which remains after the red cells and some other constituents have been removed. This is what was used principally in wartime. The patients—troops—were healthy young men who were wounded. Giving them plasma restored, at least in part, the proper total volume. Proteins and minerals were replaced. The major purpose in these cases was to prevent shock, and it is hard to calculate how many thousands of lives were saved.

Use of plasma instead of whole blood has a number of advantages: It can be kept for longer periods than whole blood; it is not vital that it be of the same type as the patient's (as I mentioned earlier, plasma ordinarily is derived from pooling blood).

Very recently, methods have been devised (and are being perfected) that permit the red cells and others to be separated from the plasma, frozen for an indefinite time, and then put back together again (reconstituted) and used. This means that donor blood, especially some of the rarer types, can be kept on hand for use at any time.

"Packed" red cells may, at times, be given (without the plasma) in instances of extreme red-cell deficiency.

Transfusions are sometimes given to people whose blood does

not clot properly, the transfused blood performing this service in the emergency. It is a temporary measure and does not permanently correct the trouble.

Indeed, transfusions do not change the patient's blood in any basic fashion. The transfusion is purely a temporary aid, although a lifesaving one. Donated red cells, for example, live only 30 to 45 days. As they gradually disappear, they are replaced by the patient's own cells. Since the matching of blood depends on the red cells, this is the explanation as to why a person's blood type cannot change as a result of a transfusion.

Some people—I've been asked many a time about this—are afraid that some error may have been made in their blood type or in keeping records. There is an excellent safeguard against this. Rarely (except for accident cases in which plasma may be used anyway) is the need for speed so great that a final and conclusive test cannot be made before a transfusion. Small samples of the patient's blood and the donor blood are mixed in the laboratory. If red cells from either tend to clump together when placed in the serum from the other blood, the transfusion is not started. Clumping is the sign of incompatibility. It is thus quite possible to tell whether the donor blood is suitable, even without knowing the types of blood involved. The incompatibility is what must be avoided.

WHEN YOU GIVE BLOOD

As we mentioned earlier, when you give a pint of blood at a blood bank (8 percent or less of your own supply) you scarcely feel its loss. It is wise to lie down and rest for half an hour afterward and to drink plenty of water or other fluids to make it easy for the body to replace the normal fluid volume. This it soon does.

Some people have an unpleasant reaction from giving blood. About all we can say is that the rest of us will have to do the giving for them.

The donor must be healthy, both for his own sake and the recipient's. It might well be, for example, that someone receiving blood from an anemic donor would come to no harm as a result of it, but he wouldn't be getting full benefit, either. And the donor would suffer from the loss of red cells he could ill afford to spare.

The more serious questions involve diseases which may be represented in the bloodstream. The important ones are syphilis, malaria and hepatitis (jaundice). Every precaution is taken to see that they are excluded.

Unfortunately, misunderstandings still occur when a patient needs blood in the hospital. Folks sometimes complain that they are charged $25 or thereabouts for a transfusion and counter belligerently, "Who's getting this money? After all, when you give blood to the Red Cross, you give it for nothing."

The answer is somewhat complicated, but it is real. First, operating a blood bank and giving transfusions is an expensive matter. It requires highly skilled people and expensive equipment. There is cost even in such things as sending a messenger to get the correct type of blood from another bank if the required type is not on hand.

Second, insistence on being paid for transfusions is a means of replacing such blood as is used. Money is one thing; blood is another. You can't manufacture blood. The only way you can get it is by having a donor give it. There is no sign that we will ever have an oversupply of it. We must be constantly on the job, reminding people that we can't save lives with transfusions unless somebody gives the blood.

There are rather vigorous disagreements in some quarters as to whether blood should be purchased from professional donors, people who use this as a money-making endeavor. When blood is thus purchased, you have to pay the fee for the blood, in addition to the cost of drawing it, keeping it, cross-matching and so on. There is, it seems to me, good reason to feel that the right way to deal with this priceless material is to give it freely as a human contribution to those around us—regardless of whether we ever know who finally uses the blood and is saved by it.

But it is likewise hard to answer the people who say, "If you can't get enough donors, how else will you get blood unless you pay for it?" The human, generous way to look at it is to expect everyone who is able to give a few pints to do so at convenient times.

To review the multiple functions of our blood: It fulfills nutritional and oxygen needs, maintains mineral balance, fights infection and is automatically equipped to prevent loss by a most efficient clotting mechanism. It is indeed the "great protector."

7

INDIGESTION FACTS AND FABLES

Maxim 7 *Take the easy road to good digestion.*

Probably no phase of health is more ridden with false ideas, old wives' tales, and either home-made or "store boughten" remedies than is the digestive process.

I can't prove it, but I wouldn't be surprised if as much "indigestion" and digestive misery is caused by folklore and lack of understanding of digestion as is caused by genuine disease.

A lot of curious beliefs have come and gone. And, unfortunately, some more of them haven't gone. When I was young, the idea of "Fletcherizing" food was popular with some people—the idea being that each mouthful of food ought to be chewed 50 times (or some other number) before being swallowed.

There have been notions, firmly cherished by some people, that certain foods (such as milk and citrus juices) shouldn't be taken at the same meal, that drinking milk in large quantities would "form a ball in the stomach" or that all of one food should be eaten first, then all of another.

All of these have had their periods of popularity and then waned, although some still survive.

Other notions, often as false and sometimes even more false, seem to go on and on. The illogical explanation of "acid stomach" is one. It is natural and, indeed, necessary for the stomach to be distinctly on the acid side. Even people who, on questioning, admit they know this, still lean on "acid stomach" as the explanation of any digestive distress.

"Indigestion" is another waste-basket term. There are real but rare cases of true indigestion. "Distress" would be a better term—but I don't mean to quarrel about terms as much as I mean to plead for a little more realization that there are a number of kinds of distress, quite unlike one another in cause, and hence requiring entirely different types of handling, if you are to expect relief.

The third big and seemingly impervious notion concerns "constipation," which is actually present in a very small number of cases supposed to be constipation—by the possessors, that is. And that will require some plain-spoken explanation a bit later.

But let's first review the basic facts of digestion—remember the humorist who once said his ambition was to write a travel book called "Down the Alimentary Canal with Gun and Camera"?

By definition, *digestion* means making food capable of being absorbed by the body tissues. The process begins about the instant food enters the mouth. Chewing is part of it, breaking up coarser foods into smaller pieces. The other part is mixing the food with saliva, especially the starches. The saliva continues its work as the food reaches the stomach and for a little time afterward, perhaps 15 or 20 minutes, after which the other digestive juices take over the work.

Let's say we're eating a ham sandwich. Bread is largely a carbohydrate of the starch family (starches and sugars are the major carbohydrates). Chewing breaks the bread into pieces, saliva moistens it and the enzyme called amylase begins breaking the starch down chemically into simple sugars, of which quite a variety exist.

The meat is primarily protein and fat. The mouth's job here is to break it up; the chemical changes will come later. The butter, margarine or mayonnaise is fat. It will wait even longer for the chemical processes of digestion to start. But we have the three major food elements: carbohydrate, protein, fat.

Shall we have some lettuce in the sandwich and add still another category? Actually, the lettuce is principally water—let a leaf of lettuce lie in the open air long enough, and it will wither away until precious little of it is left.

The value of lettuce (and other leafy vegetables) is mainly its vitamin and mineral content, which isn't large. The body needs them only in very small amounts, however. Aside from these and the water, there is a small amount of cellulose, or vegetable fiber, which will not be absorbed by the body but will provide a little bulk (residue).

Anyway, now we've eaten the ham sandwich. In small bits, it has been swallowed into the esophagus and moves on down into the stomach. With a churning action the stomach continues the process of breaking up the food and, in addition, mixing it very thoroughly with the gastric juices. Prominent among the juices are the enzyme pepsin, which begins transforming protein into a final form to be absorbed, and rennin, which curdles milk. The process of digesting fat is, to some extent, begun.

Likewise busy, breaking up the food, is hydrochloric acid. This is precisely the same acid which, in concentrated form, would burn our skin badly. In the stomach, however, it is in very dilute form. For another thing, it comes in contact with tissues that are designed by Nature to withstand its action. There must, after all, be a reason why we can digest beefsteak, yet not digest our own stomachs. This is it: a different type of tissue.

By the time our ham sandwich is ready to leave the stomach, it has been reduced to a milky, fluid mass—pretty much the consistency of gruel. If too large a chunk remains, the outlet of the stomach will choke off and close. The chunk will then be carried away from that point by the churning activity, to be further broken up. When small enough, it will pass, via the duodenum, into the small intestine.

Here, for the most part, the process of absorbing the nutrients of our food begins—alcohol is one of the few substances that is absorbed to any substantial degree by the stomach itself.

Digestive juices from the pancreas are added: trypsin for proteins, more amylase for starches, lipase for fats. Bile furnished by the liver, some directly and some by way of the reservoir called the gall bladder, co-operates in digesting fats.

By rhythmic contractions and relaxations the intestine moves the food along, the nutrients gradually being absorbed through the walls of the intestine. Most of the water is removed, too. The bulk or ash—the unusable remainder—progresses into the bowel until it reaches the rectal area. Its presence there sets up the "defecation reflex," and the waste is discharged.

WHAT REALLY IS INDIGESTION?

Indigestion is a difficult word to define. The dictionary will give you something like "imperfect digestion." That isn't what one could call specific.

Medically, true indigestion is rare. Occasionally someone may throw up undigested food, in the sense of food swallowed but unable to pass out of the stomach.

An absence of bile can interfere with, although not wholly prevent, digestion of fats. Lack of hydrochloric acid (a problem sometimes encountered by older people) hampers digestion.

There can be malabsorption problems. Cystic fibrosis is an example of a difficult disease in which the patient has to eat a great deal of food in order to absorb enough. But this is a matter of absorption rather than, strictly speaking, digestion.

The natural mechanism of the body, except in very unusual cases, is so nearly perfect that we can digest what we eat. Indigestion is hardly worth talking about except in specialized problems. So what does it mean, really, when something or other is touted as "an aid to the digestion," or when someone complains that he has indigestion? Not much.

"I've been bothered with indigestion for years," a reader says in a letter, "and have tried just about every remedy I can find in the drug store. Some of them help for a little while but then they lose their effect and the indigestion comes back as bad as ever. What can I take that will help me? I just don't know which way to turn."

A good many self-styled "indigestion" sufferers, I've noticed, are at least husky, and a lot of them are downright fat. They've been digesting a lot of food, obviously. What they really mean is that they suffer discomfort, heartburn, cramps, sharp pain, bloating, "gas" (flatulence)—I was amused by the language one woman used, seeking to be nice and not say either "belch" or "pass gas." This is the way she put it: "I am troubled with flatulence and nothing seems to help. The only thing that gives me relief is to go ahead and flatulate."

Wryly amusing as this may be, disturbances of the digestive tract mount into an enormous amount of suffering. Sometimes people add to their own misery by taking the very things they assume to be good for them. And most certainly much of the continued distress stems directly from the fact that people too often don't seek an answer to this question: What really ails me?

Hardly anyone genuinely needs to "take something to aid the digestion." The foremost exceptions may be giving very dilute hydrochloric acid when that is lacking, or the use of medications to make up for lack of bile. Even in the latter instance, however, moderate care in selection of foods and eating more frequent, smaller meals frequently proves to be a better answer. Some digestive enzymes in concentrated form can be administered if necessary.

But if such troubles as pain, cramps, gas, bloating or other unpleasant symptoms develop, the answer isn't "digestion pills." The answer is to find out what really is wrong, and then do something about it.

So shall we talk about the principal things to watch out for?

Two Kinds of Ulcers

Peptic ulcers are one of the commonest types of serious digestive ailments. Some estimates indicate that as high as one out of eight or ten people suffer from this ailment at some time, men about four times as often as women.

It is common to speak of them as "stomach ulcers," but by far the majority are in the duodenum, or outlet from the stomach. Ulcers in the stomach proper are gastric ulcers—and of the two types, the gastric ulcer is by far the more dangerous, since a high proportion of cancers are found associated with them.

Whether the gastric ulcer leads to cancer, or whether (as some authorities suspect) many gastric ulcers are merely a side effect of the beginning of cancer is to some extent beside the point. What is to be kept in mind is that the danger exists and that gastric ulcers are not to be taken lightly. If they are not removed surgically, they should be watched very carefully for any sign of malignancy. Not all gastric ulcers are cancerous—but the danger is one to be alert to.

The duodenal ulcers, on the other hand, extremely rarely have any connection with cancer. They are a painful nuisance and in some instances can be dangerous—but from another standpoint, the danger of bleeding or of perforation.

From time to time I am asked, "But, doctor, exactly what is an ulcer?" It is simply a sore, a raw place, a break in the membrane. We would call an ulcer on a finger a "sore." In the duodenum (or in the stomach) it is the same, except that the type of tissue is different, a mucous surface.

On the finger, we would treat the ulcer, at least in part and perhaps entirely, by preventing irritation and letting it heal. Basically, we try to do the same thing with a peptic ulcer—reduce irritation and let it heal itself. But since the digestive system has to be at work every day, this is not as easy to do as it is with a sore finger. There is the further complication that the ulcer, once started, is irritated by the acidulous digestive juices.

The answer, therefore, is to avoid foods that are irritating and, indeed, to use food as a shield or buffer for the ulcer. A bland diet, without irritating spices or condiments, is a basic part of the treatment. Most ulcer diets put heavy emphasis on milk, half-and-half, or cream.

In addition, a glass of milk or an even more substantial snack at strategic times between meals can amount to being a shield against irritation that develops when the stomach has been emptied, leaving the ulcer unprotected against the flow of juices.

Another source of irritation is motility, the natural movement of the digestive tract. With some people, essentially the tense, nervous person, this activity is more persistent than with others.

These are the people who can't sit still. This trait applies to more than their outward activity. At times drugs to reduce this excessive motility may be helpful.

Fortunately, this action, like all of the body processes, slows down during the sleeping hours. So does the flow of digestive juices. An active ulcer, however, can awaken the patient in the night with pain. Milk or other bland food snacks relieve this distress. Since the presence of food almost always stops the pain of a duodenal ulcer, eating a decent breakfast may well carry the patient through most of the morning.

Lunch carries him through most of the afternoon, dinner through the evening. Where necessary, milk or other snacks can be strategically timed to prevent before-lunch pain or late-afternoon pain. Depending on when the patient relaxes and goes to bed, an evening snack or a glass of milk may be required just before retiring.

The length of time between the end of a meal and the beginning of pain is not totally predictable, so schedules have to be pretty much custom-fitted to the patient. His habits, his emotions, his physical make-up, the amount he eats—all have a bearing.

In general, duodenal ulcers do not become painful until much later after a meal than is the case with gastric ulcers. This, indeed, is an important diagnostic consideration. The person with a duodenal ulcer may remain comfortable for 3 or 4 hours after a meal, yet one with a gastric ulcer may have the gnawing or burning pain start as soon as half an hour after a meal.

Exactly what causes these ulcers is something of a mystery. There are cases on record of infants having them; in such instances we must assume some constitutional weakness.

Although we cannot ascribe a specific cause, we do know with certainty about some of the things that irritate ulcers and keep them going. In fact, it might not be too feeble a thought to suggest that perhaps we all may have occasional tiny ulcers from miscellaneous trifling causes but we heal so rapidly that we have no discomfort, just as the incidental scratches that we acquire don't amount to much. Not, that is, unless some little scratch does *not* heal promptly and easily, and becomes an ulcer.

Whether this theory I have just outlined is correct isn't really, very important. It *does,* however, seem to fit with the practical facts of ulcer cases. People *do* get over ulcers, with medical help. They *stay* free of ulcers if, by then, they have learned how to treat them. That is, for practical purposes, the patient who modifies his habits so that his ulcer heals is the person who isn't likely to have any more ulcers.

But the patient who expects some sort of therapy to do it all and refuses to change his way of life, is the patient who is most difficult to treat and the one who most surely will be back again later with the same trouble.

Perhaps this letter from an annoyed ulcer patient will tell the story more clearly:

> Dear Doctor:
>
> Isn't there some more permanent method of treating a duodenal ulcer than just diet and a few pills? I have struggled through the miserable experience several times, and now the same trouble is back again.
>
> My doctor has refused to operate, but I am sure that it would be worth it to be rid of this ulcer for good instead of having it flare up every few months or so. In the long run it would be worth the time in the hospital, too.

There in a nutshell is the story of a man who may, indeed, have to have surgery eventually, and who will, most certainly, keep on having ulcer trouble, no matter what his treatment, until or unless he learns something about himself.

We know that irritating foods are bad for an ulcer. We know that irregular meals, especially with longer-than-usual lapses between eating, will be harmful. We know that highly spiced and seasoned foods irritate. We know that smoking, whether by inciting heavier flow of digestive juices or other consequences, is bad for ulcers. So is excessive alcohol. Excess acid secretion and perhaps certain drugs may be irritating.

We know very definitely that the emotional make-up of the patient is important.

A typical ulcer patient is a young, aggressive male. Whether he is a young executive fighting to go higher, or a man whose goal may be relatively modest, the overintentness with which he keeps driving is the measure of his tension.

Too much smoking, perhaps too many martinis, long hours, inadequate rest, irregularity of eating and sleeping, the refusal to take reasonable vacations—or the inability to relax when he does—are all by-products that keep his ulcer inflamed.

Go back for a moment to the letter from the man who demanded some sort of permanent cure, even surgery.

Read between the lines and you find an impatient man, one who hasn't taken the time to analyze what his treatment really amounts to, who demands perfection in the sense that it's up to somebody else to cure him.

He won't relax. He keeps on going through the ulcer treatments, which he resents and considers distasteful, and of only temporary help. His reward will be more ulcers.

If we can get such a patient to take stock of himself, assess his own habits, and revise them, then we are on the road to success. Why the rush? What's the hurry? Is all the worry accomplishing anything? Can't he do as good a job in his work if he adopts a calmer attitude, learns to relax a bit, isn't so insistent that he and everyone around him have immediate and perfect answers for everything?

One of the most telling examples of this is the hard-driving business man who gets away from his job to go hunting or fishing. He gets away from the telephone, from the details of his job, from business letters and answers. He eats anything while on this trip. His diet goes overboard. He may even indulge in too much liquor. But he relaxes—and in spite of hell and high water his ulcer calms down, too!

I've seen this happen too many times not to believe that emotional tension is, by far, the greatest single consideration in getting rid of ulcers. Yet I see people grudgingly following their diets, taking pills, following all the rules of ulcer treatment except one: Refusing to relax. And I see them continuing to suffer.

AND A FEW OTHER POINTERS

If I've convinced even one ulcer sufferer of the importance of being calm and easing the tension, then I've accomplished a good deal with the last few pages. There are a few other pointers to offer on one phase and another.

First, antacids, by counteracting the gastric juices, in some cases give ulcer patients relief. A glass of milk at the right time might do the job as well, but the patients have discovered that, for them at least, an antacid in tablet or other form subdues or eases the pain. They keep on using it, often not realizing that they have an ulcer.

You see, some ulcers are unmistakable because they are painful enough to drive the patient to the doctor promptly. Others become painful only at times, and some are known as "silent ulcers," meaning that they give no symptoms at all—but may suddenly become acute.

It is typical of ulcers to bother the possessor in streaks. Spring and fall, for whatever reason, bring more flare-ups than the other seasons. It is also common for an ulcer to be painful for a period of weeks or months, then subside for perhaps an even longer time. But with each recurrence, the following time of ease tends to become shorter.

Some ulcers remain pretty much on the surface. Others may become "craters" as they erode through the lining. If they happen to strike one of the blood vessels in the lining, there can be bleeding; whether it is light or heavy depends on the blood vessel and degree of erosion. Small but continued bleeding can cause anemia. Heavy bleeding, of course, is an immediate danger and must be treated without delay. So must a case of perforation, when the crater penetrates clear through the intestine and the threat of infection is immediate and drastic.

Thus my plea to every reader is to take seriously the task of curing ulcers early, and to avoid the perils of advanced cases. This can usually be accomplished if the patient will do his part, learn to keep his emotional turmoil at low ebb and exercise at least moderate caution after an ulcer has healed. Going back to the bad old ways of wild nerves, incautious eating, carelessness about rest, regularity and moderation as soon as an ulcer is cured is an invitation to more trouble.

As to surgery, yes, sometimes it is necessary, but it is not a cure-all. If the patient, afterward, is wise enough to maintain good habits, removal of a large and intractable ulcer can be the end of his problem. But if he does not, there is no way to insure that new ulcers will not form. There is no substitute for learning the simple rules of conservative treatment.

WHAT HEARTBURN MEANS

Heartburn, specifically, is a burning sensation underneath the breastbone. It is intense and sometimes stubborn, depending upon which of the possible causes is at work.

It may be the result of spasm of the lower part of the esophagus, the passageway through which food reaches the stomach. (The esophagus, or gullet, is in general a rugged, disease-resistant organ although esophagitis, or inflammation of it, is occasionally found.) Regurgitation of digestive juices up into the esophagus may cause heartburn.

Sometimes gall bladder disease is responsible.

Too much smoking is a known factor in heartburn.

So is nervous tension. The hard-pushing, intense person, likely to be tired at dinner time, is a prime candidate for heartburn. If he can learn to relax before meals and can cut down on his smoking, he often finds that he has achieved the answer.

Heartburn is rather common in the early months of pregnancy. And on rarer occasions, some organic disease may produce pressures that bring on the same trouble.

To boil it all down: Anxiety, pressure, nerves, haste, lack of relaxation are the most frequent culprits. If one of the more serious underlying ailments is present, this will become apparent.

But I ask you, isn't the obvious answer to try relaxing, putting haste and business concern and worry out of your mind deliberately for a time before dinner? *Try* it. It will do more than all the pills and digestion remedies you can buy.

Before we leave this topic there is one serious warning that must be voiced. In some cases, severe "indigestion" or "heartburn" can be difficult to distinguish from a heart attack. When a really severe attack occurs, the safe thing is to call the doctor. If it is a heart attack, this may mean saving a life, because the doctor can take charge at once. And if it isn't—well, perhaps your doctor can emphasize with his counsel the advice I have just offered.

A HERNIA WITH A LOT OF NAMES

A typical letter to me:

> I have been told I have a hiatus hernia, a portion of the stomach has come up into the esophagus through the diaphragm. I have never heard of such. What causes it? How can a diaphragm tear?

> R.A.

A hernia or "rupture" is a gap in some restraining "wall" of the body. The common type of hernia is in the abdominal wall. The hiatal hernia, however, is a somewhat different type. It is known also as hiatus hernia, esophogeal hernia (although that term actually should be reserved for something else), diaphragmatic hernia, chest hernia or "upside-down stomach." There may even be other names for it.

Anyway, since the diaphragm is in the way, the esophagus has to go directly through it. Now suppose the aperture through which it passes becomes slightly enlarged. It doubtless is not "torn," as the letter writer suggests; "stretched" might be a somewhat closer term.

Anyway, a varying portion of the upper part of the stomach can force its way into or through this aperture. Consequences can be anything from difficulty in swallowing to heartburn, to bleeding and the symptoms of an ulcer.

Treatment is very much like that for an ulcer—bland diet, perhaps antispasmodic drugs or other medications. Plus one other: Weight reduction many times is an excellent solution, since loss of abdominal fat reduces the pressure tending to force the stomach upward. In severe cases, surgery may be advisable and affords excellent results. Obviously, if the simpler and more conservative treatments succeed, there is no reason for surgery.

This ailment is far more frequent than the average person supposes, but doctors are very much on the alert, looking for it when other answers do not quite fit the symptoms.

FLATULENCE—LET'S CALL IT "GAS"

There's no point in denying that "gas on the stomach" may, occasionally, actually be gas. The truth is that most of it is just plain air. This is quite unbelievable to many a person who complains of "gas," but it has been proved scientifically, and perhaps I can offer some close-to-home proof, too.

Some research people have gone so far as to trap the "gas" from chronic burpers and analyze it in the laboratory. The answer? Air! Swallowed air! I remember as a youngster in my teens, going to a concert with my uncle. A few rows behind us was a chronic belcher. After 40 years I can still hear her rhythmic burps. True, gall bladder or even stomach disease can cause such trouble, but after these many years I am convinced that in her case the regularity of her burpy counterpoint came from but one cause: She was an habitual air swallower.

For a more commonplace example, what about the baby who has just had his bottle? Burping him is standard practice. Tuck him up on your shoulder, pat his back—he burps. Usually he does it without the patting.

This isn't "gas." It is air he has swallowed with his milk. In some countries in which manners depart from ours, some lusty burps are (or used to be) the courteous proof that one has enjoyed dinner. It is no accident that among such people it is proper to eat "windmill fashion," scooping food into the mouth at a fast clip. That helps them swallow enough air to provide enough belches to be polite.

Heavy beer drinkers often have considerable flatulence. Gall bladder disease may be responsible. Indeed, flatulence is one of its symptoms. Constipation, forcing material to remain more or less stationary, may permit excessive fermentation and, in that case, lead to real gas.

Allergy cannot be ignored. Some of us are, indeed, hypersensitive to certain foods. Baked beans are notorious for causing "gas" but perhaps not rightly so, as the idea has been advanced by some authorities that if the beans are not cooked with pork fat, they are far less likely to be a noisy nuisance.

By and large here are the rules for the complaint of "gas":

1. Rule out gall bladder or real stomach disease.

2. If they are not present, then eat more slowly. Watch yourself closely to see that you have not acquired, without realizing it, the habit of swallowing little gulps of air.

3. Keep the bowels regular.

If, sometimes, all of these fail, preparations containing silicone are available, the purpose being to help disperse the gas into smaller bubbles that can escape quietly.

THE "NERVOUS STOMACH"—GASTRITIS?

As I've tried to indicate, "indigestion" or other vague terms don't really get us anywhere. Neither does "nervous stomach." *We* may be nervous and overwrought, and our stomachs may respond by misbehaving. But the stomach isn't nervous of its own accord.

There is such a thing as gastritis, however, the inflammation of the lining of the stomach itself. Some authorities count it the most frequent of all stomach disturbances, and that may be. We may have only an occasional touch of it, or it may become chronic. Poisons of any sort, sometimes drugs, often tainted food can cause gastritis. And so can overeating—too much food, even if every bite of it is perfectly good.

In acute cases, one of the first signs is a feeling of fullness and nausea. There often is gas, and belching it does not allay the feeling of illness. The patient loses his desire to eat, is tired, may have a headache and even fever. Vomiting usually brings relief. There may be diarrhea.

Here again pills and potions are not of much help, but proper diet (sometimes simply eating less) usually will help.

For gastritis which results from serious poisoning, such measures as lavage, or washing out the stomach, may be required. Such cases require the attention of a physician, and I won't get into that phase as it doesn't have a great deal to do with our present purpose, which is acquiring knowledge of how to live healthy lives.

APPENDICITIS AND DIVERTICULOSIS

There is no excuse, these days, for death from appendicitis.

No particular mode of life will automatically prevent appendicitis, but everyone should know the characteristic signs of an attack. Therein lies safety.

The pain is sudden, usually, although not invariably, in the upper abdomen and the pit of the stomach, just below the breastbone. Nausea and vomiting follow in most cases. The pain settles in the lower right part of the abdomen and the abdomen is tender.

When this combination of symptoms occurs, call the doctor. An ice pack, in the meantime, may give a sense of relief, although it does nothing to help the main trouble, that inflamed appendix.

Perforation or "bursting" of the appendix is the critical danger, carrying with it the risk of peritonitis and death unless treated expertly and at once—and even then the patient must be lucky. The acute appendix needs to be removed before this happens.

Tuck the symptoms away in the back of your mind, and don't forget them. There isn't too much else you can do, but if you get medical help at once when appendicitis strikes, you have little to fear. The person who hesitates or decides, "I'll be better tomorrow" is the one in danger.

Another thing to know about but not worry about unless it makes itself known is diverticulosis.

It is quite common for small outpouchings to develop, usually in the colon but sometimes elsewhere in the digestive system. Present estimates are that 5 percent of all of us have these outpouchings, or *diverticula*. After 40 the percentage rises as age increases, until it reaches perhaps 25 to 30 percent or higher among the elderly.

Having a diverticulum means you have diverticulosis. It does not mean that you should be concerned about it. Vast numbers of diverticula exist without doing any harm or causing any symptoms, let alone discomfort or pain, and are frequently discovered only because X rays are being made for some other purpose.

The only precautions are to keep the stool soft and prevent constipation—which ought to be done anyway—and to avoid heavy intake of gross roughage foods, such as corn, nuts, bran.

The diverticulosis becomes of consequence if it progresses to another stage, diverticulitis, the *itis* ending denoting inflammation. This can result in spasm of the colon and pain or cramps, and the spasm in turn can contribute to constipation and altered bowel habits.

Severe attacks may in some ways simulate appendicitis. There may be bleeding if the irritation is excessive. In these cases specific care is necessary. A low-residue diet (to prevent physical irritation of the inflamed area), rest, analgesics to control discomfort and antibiotics to subdue infection are the usual essentials.

A large proportion of cases, once corrected, give no further trouble. Of those that do, some may eventually require surgery, but these are in the minority.

The amazing thing about diverticulitis, it seems to me, is the enormous percentage of patients who exclaim with bewilderment when they learn their trouble, "Why, I never even heard of it." These few paragraphs are my effort to see that a few more hear about it in advance and are not unduly alarmed.

COLITIS, COLITIS AND COLITIS!

> Dear Doctor:
>
> What causes colitis? And can it be cured? Especially if one is 50 years old? Can you give me some remedies for it, also diet?
>
> *Mrs. R.Y.*

I'm sure that Mrs. R.Y. expected me to reply with a flat statement of a cause for her colitis and a prescription for some not-too-unpleasant medicine that would bring all her troubles to a prompt stop. Yet to give her any kind of a single answer I would have to reply, "What kind of colitis are you talking about?" Or, indeed, it is often necessary to start off by asking a colitis patient: "What makes you think you have colitis?" For colitis, like some other ailments we've discussed, is a handy, unspecific word that is used to apply to everything from bellyache to diarrhea.

There are several major types of colitis. What helps one may be of no help with another—a thought that keeps appearing in this volume because it is so frequently true of so many things.

Mucous colitis: This is usually found in the thin, nervous individual. Transient spasm of segments of the colon is probably the best description of what really is happening, and the question is: What causes the spasms?

Direct inspection of the colon usually shows it to be normal from the organic sense, yet the patient is miserable. Mucous discharge may be found in the stool, which tends to be loose and watery because of excessively frequent activity of the bowel.

There is vague abdominal discomfort, gas, distension, aching, cramps and soreness.

In some cases the cause is food allergy, and tracing down the offending foods and eliminating them from the diet is the successful answer. In other cases, allergy seems to play no part—but the patient's nerves and habits do. Sedation, fostering a calmer attitude toward life (just as with ulcer patients), finding some way of preventing the patient from thinking and brooding so much about his belly, antispasmodic drugs to reduce activity, and a reasonably bland, balanced diet serve others well. If you can get the patient quieted and comfortable, and then the trouble starts up again in the midst of some subsequent emotional turmoil, it can be a blessing in disguise. It can illustrate vividly how large a part the emotions can play.

Ulcerative colitis: This is quite another matter, due as a rule to infection. Stool is bloody and watery. Pain and fever are present. Direct examination of the colon discloses ulcers.

Treatment here consists of bed rest, antibiotics and bland diet.

Amebic colitis: This disease is very similar to the other types of colitis, but its direct cause is the presence of a parasite rather than a germ-borne infection. Treatment is much the same except that laboratory examination of stool specimens is necessary to identify the parasite and select the proper medication to drive it off.

Irritable colon or unstable colon: Like the first type, this may be very difficult to treat, even though it is far from the most dangerous. This cannot be called "colitis" technically, because there is no inflammation or infection. It is simply a matter of the individual, doubtless without realizing it, becoming too obsessed with the "need" for frequent bowel activity, or through some other configuration of emotional tensions, having a bowel (colon) that instead of doing its work calmly and efficiently breaks into frequent flurries of activity.

Some of these patients actually cause the trouble themselves by dosing themselves with cathartics in the mistaken belief that this is necessary for health. They end up by doing their health no good and, on the negative side of the ledger, irritate and overstimulate the colon until that poor organ loses all chance of operating in normal rhythm. Take the laxatives and cathartics away from these people (no easy task, sometimes, if you are dealing with someone brought up from childhood to be bowel movement conscious) and the "colitis" begins to subside within a matter of days.

And that brings us to one more widespread problem—or at least a great many people think it is.

WRONG NOTIONS ABOUT CONSTIPATION

I do not, certainly, deny that such a thing as constipation exists. It does. But there is far less than the number of complaints would indicate. And besides that, an enormous amount of what passes for constipation can be corrected in a week or two, or perhaps sometimes a month, if people understood it better.

Any physician, I am sure, is more gratified at having a patient say, "I followed your advice and it worked," than to have a patient say, "That medicine you gave me cured me."

Why? Because it's easy to tell a patient to take a pill so many times a day, and to have him do it. It is vastly harder to persuade a patient to change his habits. That's human nature. But when you can persuade him, and he finds that your advice really works, you've accomplished a more difficult task.

One letter pleased me particularly. It was from a man who said, "I had been troubled with constipation for years. Then I began following your advice. It was only a little more than a week and the trouble stopped, and I haven't had any more since."

I've found, however, that mighty few people will take the advice unless I take the time to explain to them why it will work.

Let's start at the beginning. What do you mean by "constipation"? Believe it or not, I once received a virulent letter from a woman who had fallen into the clutches of one of the quack cults and who bawled me out for disagreeing with her "doctor" who had persuaded her that "unless you have at least six bowel movements a day, it is the worst kind of constipation."

How such utter rubbish can be believed is beyond me. And you. Yet some people fall for it. If they keep up the quack programs of enemas, cathartics, straining in the bathroom, and overeating of too much bran or other scratchy forms of bulk, in the end they stand an excellent chance of becoming chronic bowel invalids. And perhaps worse.

So what *is* constipation? What may be normal regularity for me may not be for you. As a general rule, one movement a day is regarded as adequate. Some people with a yen for foods with a lot of bulk—and I have no quarrel with such people, if they like it—sometimes find a second movement necessary.

For others and they are perfectly healthy, it may be once every two to four days. I had a skinny uncle who went once a week and didn't worry about it. He was sufficiently happy, active and long-lived, as well as reasonably free from diseases, that I can't think of any reason why he shouldn't have done just as he did. He went to the bathroom when Nature told him to, and that was fine.

Yet many people go into a panic if they do not have a bowel movement once a day (or in the case of the fanatics, more often). They rush for the laxatives, force the colon to empty itself, then start worrying why they can't repeat the process the next day.

It takes perhaps two to three days for the forcefully emptied colon to accumulate enough waste to cause the "defecation reflex." So what do they do? Grab for the laxatives again, forcing the colon into needless activity and perhaps bringing about a small movement which might better have waited until the proper time.

This is not constipation. This is idiocy.

Real constipation is quite a different thing. The lean individual with ptosis (or low position of intestinal structure) may occasionally be troubled with constipation.

The old person, a light eater and physically inactive, and particularly the elderly bed-patient, may quite often become constipated. Wastes do not accumulate very rapidly, and as they wait for enough to trigger the reflex that will expel them, they become dried, hardened—impacted.

Obstructions, whether from congenital fibrous bands or adhesions from an operation, can impede normal movement. Kinking or narrowing of the bowel at some point may be present. Poor muscle tone of the gut sometimes is found.

But for all of these causes, more constipation is man-made. Much, as already indicated, is because some folks (too many!) have been brought up to be bowel-fussers. From childhood they have been told that they must have a movement at least once a day. If they didn't, they were forced to take laxatives or have enemas. Result: The bowel, never left to adopt a normal rhythm, perpetually is forced to respond to purges.

Along with this is the notion of "colonic irrigation" or "high colonic," which is a fancy term for an enema. Sure, enemas have their uses, but a healthy person doesn't often need them. The net result of these "colonic irrigations" is to foul up the natural working of the colon and produce artificial constipation for two or three days afterward because there hasn't been time for a normal movement to follow.

Faulty eating and drinking (and by the latter I mean not getting enough fluid) is a second major cause. If we absorbed everything we ate, there would be nothing to discharge. In practice this is an impossibility, but the amount of ash or residue varies quite considerably from one food to another. Bran, for example, the hard shell-like covering of grains, contains almost no nutritional elements that we can absorb. Corn, sweet and tender as it may be in the sweet-corn season, contains a considerable amount of similar undigestible "shell" material. After all, corn is a form of grain. The fibers of oranges and other fruits and vegetables are in the same category. They are bulk, not food.

For regularity we need a certain amount of bulk, and most of us get it in our normal meals. If we don't, then bulk producers—psyllium seed, agar and plantage preparations are very useful. The older person who is inactive and doesn't need as much food for energy is often helped by these. Besides, the older person may, perhaps because of trouble with teeth or for other reasons, not eat as much of the foods containing natural bulk.

Insufficient water intake is another cause of constipation. I cannot stress this too much. If there is some moderate slowness of bowel activity and the fecal matter hardens, then a hurtful aspect of constipation arises. It becomes physically difficult to move this hardened mass.

Time after time the mere insistence that a constipation victim drink more water has been a most successful treatment. If this is sweetened or flavored water, it is still fluid. Tea, coffee, fruit juices, lemonade—all are good. Prune juice is *very* effective.

Many people swear by the idea of the juice of half or all of a lemon in a glass of water in the morning. I have no objection whatever—although I know others who drink plain water and fare as well. (The lemon juice, however, is a good source of Vitamin C.) Some want warm water. Others use tap water. It's still water!

A good rule of thumb for the person having trouble with hardness is to drink a glass of water on arising, another in midmorning, one in midafternoon and another in the evening. Four glasses of water, in addition to whatever is consumed at meals or just because you are thirsty, can make a world of difference. And has.

Where for one reason or another the patient, say a bed-bound invalid, may rebel at drinking this much fluid, an alternative recourse is in the use of dioctyl sodium sulfosuccinate, a chemical known as a softening agent, which makes the greatest possible use of such moisture as is available in the system. It is sold under a dozen or so different trade names.

Finally, responding to the call of Nature, the urge to go to the bathroom, is important. Heed it, and things proceed normally. Put it off, and the human system, like a pouting child, reacts as though saying, "You wouldn't when I wanted to, so now I'll just sulk."

Silly way to acquire constipation, isn't it? But as human beings we are perverse. We do it. And we suffer for it. So if you have a sincere desire to overcome constipation, don't resist the natural urge. You will soon find yourself falling into an habitual pattern of going at some particular time, perhaps after breakfast or at some other time of day. If your problem has been severe and sometimes you get no results at the usual time, a glycerin suppository can help. Don't think you will always need it. You won't. But it will help establish the pattern.

Likewise, give yourself at least some minutes of leeway. Sit, relax, keep a magazine or book handy. But let that natural rhythm become a regular habit.

I've talked more people out of constipation than I have treated out of it. There's a reason. Constipation isn't natural. Regularity is. Constipation isn't a disease. It is a departure from normal.

You may ask whether a laxative ever is necessary, on the basis of what I've just said. Occasionally, yes. More often, merely helpful. If you've gotten out of the pattern of regularity and need some help, use either natural laxatives or the milder chemical ones. Eat a couple of oranges instead of settling for juice. (The bulk will help.) Or a dish of prunes, or some prune juice. Very good laxatives.

Avoid harsh laxatives, such as epsom salts or castor oil, which empty the bowel too completely. They require you to wait too long before normal action can resume.

Milk of magnesia is a milder one. So is cascara, but I would caution against taking more of it than the directions recommend. Enough is fine. Too much becomes irritating. Mineral oil is a good lubricant. Too frequent or continued use, we are told, interferes with absorption of Vitamin A. This, however, has not been conclusively proved. An occasional spoonful isn't going to hurt anything and often does the trick.

The goal, always, is to get back to normal.

8

PREVENT MENTAL BREAKDOWN

MAXIM 8 *Nip mental illness early. As with most physical illnesses, treatment is usually very effective when the illness is just starting. Allowed to go on untreated, it can become chronic and disastrous.*

Probably the shortest letter I've ever received relating to this problem follows in full:

> Dear Dr. Molner:
>
> Would you please explain the difference between mental illness, insanity and crazy? Gratefully,
>
> *M.B.C*

It's as good a place to start as any.

If I could have just one wish in this matter of mental health, I would wish that the words *insanity* and *crazy* could be scrubbed out of the language as though they never had existed, and the general attitude that brought the words would disappear just as completely.

Crazy is a wastebasket word, into which we dump any sort of inexact meaning that we can't (or won't take the trouble to) express more precisely. It can mean that a person has been in a mental hospital. It may mean that he does things in unusual ways, or that we disagree with his judgment. Or we say, "I'm crazy about him (or her)," and we mean something quite different. The word *crazy* means anything or nothing.

Insanity is another matter—but it is a word I would like to get rid of. From the medical or psychiatric standpoint, it doesn't mean anything. It is strictly a legal term. It means what a court and jury decide it means. There is no absolute definition of it. The dictionaries offer such phrases as "of unsound mind."

But when you stop to think of it, what is the exact definition of *sick* or *well*? Again there is no exact dividing line—as is shown clearly enough when somebody decides whether to go to work or stay home.

One fellow will explain that he has a bad cold, headache, upset stomach and is "too sick to go to work." Another, who wants to go to work, will take his drippy nose to his job, exposing his fellow workers to his particular virus, but he figures that he is "well." Or well enough to go to work, anyway.

Where do you draw the line? If you have a sore toe, are you well? Not completely. But are you sick?

So it is with mental health. The exact line is impossible to define but depends on judgment. Just being nervous, or having some oddity of behavior, doesn't mean that a person is mentally ill. And on the other hand, some inmates of mental hospitals behave just as reasonably as anyone on the outside. I have particularly in mind a man who, so long as he was in the hospital, was sane by any sort of test or examination or observation the lawyers might choose to apply.

He was allowed to leave the hospital, go downtown or anywhere else that an errand might demand, and he never got into any trouble. In the hospital he took charge of entertainment programs for his fellow patients, and in this regard he was just about the equivalent of an extra staff member.

But when he was discharged from the hospital, it took only a week or two for him to crack up emotionally. He would promptly worry himself into such a state that he couldn't do any work, couldn't make up his mind about the ordinary problems of living. Pretty soon he would be back in the hospital. There he would regain his composure and ability to do an excellent job of living.

He is as good an example as I can think of, of the person who needs to be constantly supported emotionally. He has to have the feeling that he is safe and protected, that he need not assume the responsibility for looking after himself—earning a living, paying his bills, getting along with those around him.

To him, the hospital was a refuge, feeding him, clothing him, lifting from his shoulders all the worries that go with living in society.

You may say that he should be taught responsibility, that he was shirking his share of the world's duties. You may feel that he must have been poorly brought up to have adopted such a feeble attitude toward life. Perhaps that is so. I do not happen to know about his childhood and youth. I do know, however, that he had managed to earn a very adequate living in a skilled, specialized line of work, until he was in his latter twenties or early thirties. He took the pressures as long as he could, and then he cracked.

A Good Word to Know

Many people directly involved in mental care use a word which is little known to the public—but ought to be. The word is *resocialized*.

There are countless patients sharing, to some degree, the problem of the man I just described. They go to a mental hospital because they have reached the point at which they cannot get along in society. With a chance to rest from their particular pressures, and with treatment by the hospital, they acquire enough emotional stamina, enough faith in themselves and sometimes some know-how concerning the world and the people in it, so they can go back to living in ordinary society. They become resocialized.

To be sure, there are some patients in the hospitals who never will be released because they never will be able to acquire what they need to become resocialized.

In hospitals for people whom we call, legally, the "criminal insane," there are some in whom hate has become such a part of their driving force that they have to be kept locked in single cells. Some are catatonic—in their resentment against the world and their determination to have nothing to do with it, they lie hour after hour without moving a muscle, as though paralyzed. The paralysis, however, is not physical. It is in their tortured minds.

There are the paranoid patients, many of whom have been extremely hard to detect. They become adroit at assuming the outward signs of a normal person. Inwardly, they are constantly plotting and constantly suspicious that others are plotting against them. Possibly we should reverse the order there; doubtless in some cases the plotting against others is the result of unending fear. It is a reaction, the desire to strike back, even though they are striking back against dangers that are wholly imaginary.

Yes, there are such patients. But they are few in comparison to the millions whose mental illnesses imply no peril to the people around them and may be of relatively brief duration.

Mike Gorman, in his splendid book, *Every Other Bed,*[*] did a great deal to make vividly clear to us the extent of mental illness. It is quite true, as his title indicates, that in the United States there are as many beds for mental patients as there are for all physical ailments combined. It has been calculated that one person in every ten will spend some time in a mental hospital and that more will require medical attention for emotional troubles.

It is frequently speculated that the tensions of modern life are responsible for a great increase in mental illness. This I am inclined to doubt. There have been pressures and tensions and fears in other ages. Our society today may be more complex, but are the anxieties any greater than they were for pioneer families who lived in fear of starvation if they could not grow enough crops? Or for city dwellers in the days of the great plagues? Or those who lived under oppressive laws that could order a child hanged for stealing a pocket handkerchief?

No, I can't agree that our anxieties today are necessarily greater than those of our ancestors. It is more likely, however, that mental illness becomes more readily identified today. Only two or three generations ago, the vast part of our society was rural or semirural. On the farms and in the small towns it was easier, I am sure, for a family to take care of Uncle Willie who "wasn't

---

* Mike Gorman, *Every Other Bed* (New York: World Publishing Company, 1956).

quite right in the head." He learned what he could or could not do, and where he might go. His eccentricities were tolerated by the comparatively few people with whom he came in contact.

In the city, and more particularly perhaps in apartment-house living, the situation is quite different. The neighbors, not understanding Uncle Willie very well, become alarmed. They are afraid he "might do something."

The complexities of jobs in modern society are such that vagaries or unreliability cannot be permitted. The overwrought individual who gives way to tears, anger or utter collapse under his pressures, fears and worries soon finds himself out of a job.

Yes, I believe that our modern society forces us to recognize more cases of emotional illness, and it demands that more treatment be available for patients.

WHAT CAUSES MENTAL ILLNESS?

Only a couple of hundred years ago it was quite firmly believed by the "authorities" that "lunacy" was caused by the moon. The "lunatics" were supposed to be thus "possessed of devils," and it was accepted treatment to beat the patients, stamp on them, whip them, half-drown them to "drive out the devils."

As little as a century ago, even in "enlightened" communities, mental hospitals (or asylums) kept patients in chains as a routine measure or sometimes kept them locked interminably in dungeons. As recently as the 1950's we have still had some shocking exposures of cruelty to mental patients by employees who didn't know better.

Today I believe and hope that these dark ages are past. Certainly I do not myself know of any hospital in which such brutalities would for a moment be permitted. If I did, I most certainly would raise a storm about it tomorrow morning—and I would have support from all directions.

We have learned at last that mental illness is just that—an illness. We have found a considerable number of ways of treating it successfully, though not every case is amenable.

But we do not know with any certainty what causes it.

There have been two schools of thought, one being that emotional trauma of some sort must be responsible. That, in other words, if this is an illness of the mind and the emotions, then mental and emotional impacts must be the cause.

Another (and growing) concept is that certain physical conditions are at the root of the trouble.

There is now, among those most knowledgeable, the conviction that both are right, and that mental illness must be a consequence of both factors. Complicated research experiments now in progress continue to support this view. It is highly logical. Granted that some people, by heredity or the workings of the body's chemistry are not able to withstand as much stress as the rest of us, why be astonished that they break down mentally under impacts which are withstood by someone else with relative ease? We all have a "cracking point." Possibly no two of us have precisely the same one.

We certainly know that these things work in reverse. We have the man mentioned early in this chapter who, relieved of emotional stresses, became by all observable symptoms emotionally well. He had low tolerance for even simple stresses.

On the other hand, we can see physical changes in many mental patients. Their manner of walking can change. They may become lethargic—or, under pressures that they cannot support, they may break into some sort of violence.

There is growing reason to believe that there are changes in the chemistry of the blood and that this, no doubt, must be reflected in many organs of the body, although the precise changes are subtle and study is extremely difficult. Still, we make progress. We don't know the whole story by any means. But we do know enough to treat most mental ailments intelligently and effectively.

WHAT GOOD ARE TRANQUILIZERS?

The ataractic drugs, or tranquilizers, burst with dramatic suddenness onto the scene. They were—and are—so effective that perhaps many of us lost sight of their real significance.

They do "tranquilize" a person, and they perhaps have been

overused by people who wanted to escape from pressure by taking a pill that would let them brush their worries aside.

This, of course, is not a truly sensible attitude toward life. A pill doesn't solve our problems, even though it can help us ignore them for the moment.

However, let's examine their usefulness in mental illness. We have been warned often enough by now that tranquilizers do not cure mental illness but are a sensationally useful tool to be used in the process.

Take the person who has just about reached his "breaking point," either because basically he has a low cracking point, or because he has been under far too much pressure far too long.

He (or she) reaches the point at which he can't take any more stress. It is a matter of the straw that broke the camel's back. Somebody makes a simple remark, but the emotionally tensed individual finds some reason to resent it and goes into a howling, clawing rage. The tantrum is all out of proportion to the incident —but it was just the final straw. It is the sort of thing that occurs in mental illness.

Or, alternatively, the patient (not yet recognized as being a patient) swallows the presumed insult, but the pressure continues to build up inside. Yes, there is a great deal to be said in favor of getting things off your chest. Let the resentment build up long enough inside, and it explodes.

The tranquilizers, by helping the patient to ignore some of his pressures and worries, bring him at least a little of the way down from his exploding point. There have been some classic instances in the last few years of people who, having reached and passed that point, did everything from smashing their own dishes and furniture to trying to fight everyone who came within arm's reach.

Only a few years ago these were the people who would have been subdued physically by the police, wrapped in strait jackets, and finally dumped into an isolation room in a hospital until time and exhaustion eased their pressures and someone could at least talk to them.

Today, if they can be persuaded to swallow a tranquilizer, they calm down and will listen to reason, at least to a useful extent. They are, obviously, in need of some treatment to help them release or control their pressures, but they stop exploding.

At one of the large mental hospitals with which I am familiar, soon after the tranquilizers had come into use, there was a complaint from the supply department of the hospital. For some reason, the head of that department complained, he wasn't getting nearly the number of torn-up sheets, pillow cases and clothing that he used to get. What was the matter? If this situation wasn't corrected at once, the hospital would have to start purchasing cleaning rags!

In this entire hospital, you see (but he didn't at first see!), the tranquilizers were keeping disturbed patients below their exploding point. They weren't going into frenzied rages of destruction. They weren't making enough rags.

The supply manager, naturally, was mightily pleased when he learned the explanation, and for years now the hospital has been buying cleaning rags (much cheaper than sheets and clothes).

More important, more of the patients have more quickly been reaching the point at which they could be resocialized—that is, go home, or out into society. The same hospital used to have a wing of one building devoted to isolation rooms into which they could put patients who became violent after going beyond the limit of their emotional tolerance. With more than 3,000 patients, this was a daily, or more frequent, occurrence.

Today only a room or two is kept in reserve for emergency. The rest of these bare, rugged, barred rooms have been curtained, painted and refurnished into rooms used only when one of the patients falls ill with a physical sickness and has to be hospitalized within the hospital for pneumonia, an ear infection, kidney stones or some such complaint.

So More Patients Go Home

The over-all result is that hospital patients need not remain hospitalized so long. They can converse with the doctors sooner. They can relax sooner. They can examine the matters which have worried them, made them angry or made them fearful.

Since some of them have been building up for most of their lives to the exploding point, this is not a rapid process. Yet the earlier they can begin to think clearly about their problems, the earlier they can find some substantial answers.

Some, on a sort of border line, can go home very quickly, because even after they leave the hospital they can keep their exploding point below the danger line by continuing to use the tranquilizers.

Obviously we cannot expect drugs alone to do it all. They are a tool. They save the borderline cases. They help the difficult ones. Mental hospitals, once crowded and pressured by hopelessly long waiting lists, are starting to catch up. The tranquilizers have been and are a wonderful help. But they can't do it all. They can't do more than a reasonable share.

The Line that Divides the "Ill"

If you ask me for some specific rule to use to identify the beginning of mental illness, I cannot give it to you.

A psychiatrist, having spent perhaps 15 years of his life getting a college, medical and finally psychiatric education, can readily identify the psychotic patient—the one whose mental illness is at or near the hospitalization level.

In industry there is growing reliance on psychology and psychiatry at the other end of the scale, for people who have never been in a mental hospital and probably never will be.

Here is an example of which I had knowledge a few years ago. An excellent workman was being considered for a supervisory job. The psychological department advised against it. The man, they said, was of an emotional make-up that would not absorb the responsibilities required in the new job.

"In 6 months," they said, "he'll be over his depth and realize it, and he'll go to pieces."

The warning was rejected. The man was known as such a "steady" chap. But things turned out just as predicted, and within a few days of the 6-month forecast, too. The man complained that he just couldn't stand another day in the new job; could he go back to his old one? He was allowed to do so, of course.

My point is that mental health is not a yes-or-no matter, like having or not having pneumonia. Rather, it represents a long, long scale of values, just as physical health does, ranging from a scratched finger to the most serious of conditions as, say, the terminal stages of cancer.

With a scratched finger we don't count ourselves as ill. If the finger becomes badly infected, then we do.

It is the same with mental health. We all have our inherent strengths and weaknesses. We are exposed to differing pressures.

For common-sense purposes, we speak of a person as being "mentally ill" when he reaches a point at which his emotional problems interfere with the affairs of his daily life—when reasonably effective family life is disrupted, when he can't do his job properly, perhaps when he can struggle along with job and family matters but is so constantly miserable, emotionally, that sooner or later something will have to "give."

When dad is harried by too many bills, and he isn't sure he won't be laid off from work, and he needs a rest but can't take it, it is perfectly understandable that he may become curt and snappish, yell at the kids and growl at his wife.

That isn't what we mean by mental illness. It is, all the same, a matter of mounting emotional tension, and how well he tolerates it is the measure of his basic emotional strength.

How One Doctor Does It

I know one doctor who, with his colleagues at a big public hospital, has had considerable success by keeping exactly this kind of thought in mind when emergency cases are brought in to the psychiatric department.

These are people who have come to their own personal exploding points, emotionally, and have behaved in such a way as to make it necessary for relatives, neighbors or the police to take them to the hospital.

They may have started breaking things, or going into uncontrollable fits of weeping, or refusing to eat, or refusing to leave their rooms, or talking incessantly and perhaps not very rationally; or they may otherwise have displayed signs that they were strongly upset. In some cases they went to the hospital voluntarily, knowing that they were reaching a condition that they could not control.

Some of these people really needed hospitalization. Others, however, needed only someone to take an interest in them, to advise them, or, to borrow a phrase from the language of this field of care, they "needed some emotional support."

The aim, in this hospital (and I fondly hope that the same goal is being adopted in quite a few others), was for the psychiatrists to talk to these patients as soon as possible after their arrival—in any event, the same day.

Endless kinds of problems bother people. They involve money, fears, worries, lack of affection, loneliness, the piling on of burdens too great to carry, obsessive fear of illness—the list could go on.

Many a time the psychiatrists, being able to take a detached view, could offer some perspective on the problem: If you do thus and so, it will simplify things. Or: This is not your problem; do your share and let other people handle the rest. Or: You've magnified this problem beyond the dimensions it deserves.

This friendly and human approach has been very useful. True, some people have gone beyond range of such elementary help before they arrive, and more substantial treatment is required before they can climb back to the level which we call being "socialized," or being able to cope with the ordinary problems of living in society.

It depends on the depth of the difficulty at the time it appears before the eyes of someone who can evaluate it. Many of the potential patients, luckily getting some help—emotionally speaking—at the right moment, have been able to get back on an even keel. Sometimes it has been such simple advice as saying, "Yes, you've had your troubles and you are behind with the rent—but if you just explain to your landlord that you've had difficulties, but you have a job and can pay him $10 on account next Tuesday, and can gradually catch up with the rest, things will straighten out."

Yes, these things have, in some cases, pushed somebody to the brink of catastrophe. It depends, of course, on the way you have been brought up, and the attitudes that you have been acquiring all your life. To some of us, being in debt just a few dollars has become a sin. Others can be in debt up to their ears, and it doesn't upset them much—but for them the feeling of "not being important" is a terribly oppressive thought. We're all different.

By any chance does this help describe the endless variety of things which weigh on our minds and emotions?

Is Nervousness Mental Illness?

Here's a letter which is pretty much typical of thousands that I have received:

> Dear Doctor M.:
>
> I would like to see an article on nervous conditions.
>
> I have that uneasy feeling in my stomach and a tight throat, and woozy feelings that lay me up and I don't feel equal to going anywhere or enjoying life.
>
> I have been to several doctors and taken treatments to relieve tension (I have nothing to worry about) but get very blue about my condition. Is there such a thing as disease of the nerves? Are there nerve specialists?
>
> I rest a lot but do not sleep well, and have that weak, tired feeling. What should one do to regain your energy and pep?
>
> *Mrs. C.P.H.*

In many ways the words "nerves" and "nervous" are deceptive.

Nerves, strictly speaking, are sensitive, intricate mechanisms that carry signals (or sensations) from one part of the body to another. They are, principally, quite automatic.

We use these long, sensitive trains of nerves to carry the signal to the muscles when we want to move a finger. We use them when it is necessary for us to be aware that our toes have been stepped on, or that we have touched a hot stove, or that we are hungry, or that a loud noise startles us.

Nerves are the telegraph system of the body, but more sensitive than any system of wires contrived by man. There are neurologists who are true nerve specialists.

Yet the word "nervous," or the phrase "I have trouble with my nerves," is quite another matter. How real nerves ever got mixed up with emotions, or the way we *feel* about things, I shall never know.

The brain is the nerve center in more ways than one. If we touch a hot stove, the nerves carry the signal to the brain and the brain sends back a signal to the muscles to move, to stop touching the hot stove. These signals travel at unbelievable speed, so the reaction is just about instantaneous—some small fraction of a thousandth of a second, perhaps, in transit.

But the "nerves" that we are considering are just carriers of messages. It is in the compact brain that we acquire such things as learning, memory, reasoning. It is in this area that we learn to look forward and backward, to fret, to fear, to be anxious.

I don't know how many times I have heard and seen the phrase, "nerve medicine." It is a faulty phrase. It may mean a sedative, a drug that is administered to slow down the whole system. It may mean a tranquilizer, a medicine which mankind has at last evolved to relax our built-in capacity to worry about things.

Yet neither can take the place of real emotional tranquility. That is something which most of us achieve, and must achieve, by our "thinking ability." I know I have not used a very good term here, but I don't know a better one.

All of us have known since childhood the tensions that derive from waiting, worrying, anticipation. For a close-to-home example, I am forever aware of a little girl who, for whatever reasons, had built up Halloween to be the most exciting holiday of the year. She looked forward to it for weeks. She fussed with her costume and mask. She had a shopping bag ready to go out begging.

She built up, and up—to a letdown.

For all the years of her little-girlhood, she invariably reached such a pitch of anticipation that late in the afternoon of her wonderful evening, she lapsed into an upset stomach and often a headache—and spent the magic hours of early evening lying on a couch feeling ill.

A tragedy of childhood? Certainly. Could we have avoided it by taking the position, from the time she was 4 years old, that Halloween was a prosaic affair, and not very exciting? I suppose so—now. But how could parents deliberately suppress the happy anticipation of a child who had selected this event as the one that excited her most?

We all know the boy who was a bundle of nerves before a football game but settled down after the first whistle. And the girl who, before her first party date, was a trembling, unsure, tearful child, afraid she would be "stood up" or wouldn't measure up. But her awkward, wonderful boy arrived with his eyes full of stars, and suddenly life was wonderful for both of them.

It is normal for us to worry and wonder. Normal for us to fear the things that warrant fear. The fool who "doesn't know the meaning of fear" usually comes to grief because of his bravado.

It is normal to be afraid of dangerous things and sensible to display a certain amount of concern over our affairs. A reasonable amount of stress in our lives not only doesn't hurt us but probably is very necessary for our well-being and total happiness.

WHEN SHOULD WE SEEK HELP?

It is quite another situation when we are beset by worries that have no basis. This is precisely what some people do. Their anxieties are vague, even though intense. They literally cannot tell what they are worrying about and, if pressed, will "explain" by mentioning trivial things or use excuses such as "my health" when there is no sign of illness, or "financial uncertainty" when they are in no difficulty.

Doubtless some fixed anxieties may be rooted in experiences early in life, not consciously remembered by the individual, or deliberately pushed aside because the memory is painful. As the emotional sensitivity or weakness of the patient is attacked by whatever frustrations, cruelties or rejections he may be encountering, there comes a point at which something has to happen.

Pent-up frustration can explode into rebellion or rage. The actual event touching off the explosion may be trivial. It is the total pressure which counts. Or the person may try to escape from his unhappiness by withdrawing. Sometimes an obsessive resort to religion occurs. Now religion is of great value to any of us—but not when someone tries to use it as an escape from reality.

Others try to submerge their cares, whether real or imagined, in alcohol or drugs, and some become swamped by excessive use of sedatives or even narcotics.

The very severe psychoses, or mental illnesses, can be interpreted as a method of escape or at least an attempt to escape from life's problems, with the patient hearing voices that nobody else hears, or having other hallucinations. Terrified fears of being pursued by foreign agents or even our own police forces are not unusual in severe cases. Or there is an obsession that "they are doing something to my mind by secret radio waves."

These deep manifestations are obvious enough, and people generally are more and more willing to call for help instead of trying to hide the growing sickness of a relative.

In the earlier stages there is no ready rule for knowing when a situation is starting to get out of hand. These matters rarely if ever develop from any single experience or incident, however shocking. They grow slowly and insidiously.

Being aware of the nature of emotional illness is our first means of protection. Next is the physician. I do not mean a psychiatrist, but rather the physician who takes care of the individual or family on a continuing basis. There is a steady increase in the number of doctors who have some added training in psychiatry beyond that which they may have received in school. The family physician is also likely to have the understanding which comes from dealing with patients over the years.

Sometimes some other trusted family counselor, perhaps a clergyman, will have a much clearer perspective of the beginning of a mental problem because he is not quite so close to it. Sometimes an employer recognizes signs which deserve professional attention.

One thing is certain: We have, in recent years, made very considerable strides. More and more general hospitals are establishing psychiatric units. Clinics and institutes are being opened for people who are not yet at the stage of needing hospitalization and can be saved from it.

With increasing success we are seeing patients who have reached the emergency state being rescued by brief but intense care in a general hospital's psychiatric section, perhaps for only a few days or a week or two, followed by office visits to guard against losing the progress that has been made.

Patients going into hospitals (usually state institutions) for long-term care are coming out again with greater regularity, and "day hospitals" and after-care clinics are preventing them, in many cases, from having to go back in. Support, encouragement and sometimes continued use of tranquilizers or other medications help the patients rebuild their emotional stamina gradually until they can go it alone again.

But let us also keep this very firmly in mind: Maintenance of mental health and mental treatment are very much more than phases of a last-ditch struggle to keep people out of hospitals. It is not inevitable that every mental disorder is bound to progress to the need for a hospital. Far from it! Most will *not*.

So let us go one step farther in trying to decide when professional attention is needed. Do so on the basis of the need to be more comfortable—which, after all, is about the same rule we use in seeking attention for physical needs, isn't it?

I cannot honestly say that I feel this to be an adequate answer for everyone. It will depend on where he lives, the availability of psychiatric care and on the extent to which his regular physician is able to assess and treat emotional problems of lesser dimensions.

We don't have enough psychiatrists, nor enough treatment centers, nor enough physicians in other fields who are capable of doing as much as we might like. The numbers of all are increasing, but the demand still far exceeds the supply.

WHAT YOUR DOCTOR CAN DO FOR YOU

In spite of these lacks, we are far ahead of our position of only a few years ago. With tranquilizers available in great variety, the personal physician can help many a patient over a particularly troubled phase. He can urge his patients to assess their own needs; the failures and frustrations are a relative matter. The most frustrated person may not be one who has achieved little. He may sometimes be the man (or woman) of great drive, ambition and competitive spirit, who has achieved a great deal but still does not consider it enough. Hence, a sort of high-level frustration.

Diet, heredity, physical make-up and physical condition all have their reflection in the emotional situation. Of these, one or two can be helped.

Another, and very widespread emotional disorder, also can be helped. This is depression. The psychiatrists can differentiate several types, but for our purposes, that is not necessary.

The symptoms are scattered: Headache, dizziness, rapid heart, loss of appetite, digestive upsets, urinary complaints and sexual impotence have all been found stemming from depression. All, of course, can arise from other causes, but when other known causes cannot be found, the answer may be depression.

Usually other signs will be apparent, among them melancholia, a tendency to blame others for whatever goes wrong, anxiety moods, self-depreciation, loss of interest in one's appearance, inability to relax, insomnia, abnormally early waking in the morning, guilt feelings, disinterest in changes—indeed, disinterest in the world in general.

Depression, besides being responsible for direct destruction of happiness and usefulness, is increasingly being recognized as a cause of suicide. Needless suicides run into the thousands. How high the total really is becomes a matter of conjecture because so many times suicide is not recognized as such or is concealed by those around the victim.

Depression most often attacks in middle age or somewhat after middle age. The outlook is rather optimistic, if the condition is recognized, and if the patient can be helped over the worst of it.

Nature tends to correct it, given time. Too often Nature does not have time. The victim takes his own life, or he is killed in what appears to be an accident. Or if not that, the period of depression may have severe impact on his life, causing loss of job, breakup of family, alienation of friends.

In the last few years drugs known as "psychic energizers" have been proving very effective in treating depression, whereas earlier, electroshock therapy often had to be used. I will not go so far as to say that electroshock may not still be preferable in some cases, but the psychic energizers have reduced the number of cases requiring it. Further, the energizers, given in tablet form or capsules, do not require that the patient be hospitalized, unless the particular case is so acute as to demand it.

Thus a whole new avenue of approach is developing in this large region of emotional disorders.

ALCOHOL—AND OTHER KINDS OF DRUGS

Alcoholism, for some victims of emotional disorders, is an escape. So are drugs. Some patients have gotten into the dangerous cycle of using sedatives to go to sleep, then using amphetamines or "pep pills" the next day to rouse themselves from oversedation.

This is a pattern which too often has led at last to the "overdose of sleeping pills" we read about. The human system cannot indefinitely support such a violent up-and-down course. Another end result is collapse of the patient, physically and emotionally.

Once launched on this perilous course, the patient should have medical help, psychiatry if possible. The same is true of those who have gotten the barbiturate habit or have become addicted to narcotics. Dependence on "pep pills" likewise is dangerous, and it is apparent that considerable illegal traffic in them is going on.

But of all the drugs, alcohol is the most prevalent. Estimates of the number of alcoholics run into the millions. There is no exact definition of alcoholism. Not everyone who takes a drink is an alcoholic—not even everyone who drinks too much for his own good.

Alcoholism is the warranted term for the condition of a drinker who becomes dependent on alcohol, feeling that he needs and must have it; his drinking begins to interfere with his normal life. This does not mean that the drinker—man or woman, and there are many more woman alcoholics than you might suppose—has to become "falling-down drunk." Many a real alcoholic never makes a spectacle of himself in public. He frequently prides himself on his ability to "hold his liquor," and he may have the same reputation among those who know him.

If he needs the liquor, depends on it, he is an alcoholic. Even if, as many alcoholics do, he "goes on the wagon" periodically, it doesn't change the situation. This is, in fact, a rather frequent pattern for alcoholics. They stop drinking for a month, or perhaps for several months, with the feeling that it proves that they can take it or leave it alone. The real proof, however, is that after this binge of sobriety, the need for alcohol catches up with them. They miss a few days at work, or do their work badly. Some can't resist sprees of spending along with their drinking, and wind up with a burden of debts to pay off.

But why describe all the different kinds of alcoholics there are? For any of them, there is only one good answer and that is to stop drinking. This they must do themselves, whether they get the help of some of the excellent alcohol clinics, or follow the principles of Alcoholics Anonymous.

Malnutrition is part of the alcoholic's lot. He may be fat or *appear* well nourished from calories of his alcohol intake but he is wanting in adequate diet. He does not eat properly when he drinks. Vitamin deficiency occurs.

The liver—the great clearing house of the digestive tract—becomes poisoned from the by-products of alcohol metabolism. It lacks protection from protein, carbohydrate or vitamins. Changes occur in the liver—cirrhosis. The ravages of this can take their toll in the alcoholic long after he has taken the pledge and gone on the wagon. Death from liver failure or massive hemorrhage resulting from cirrhosis is not uncommon.

Brain damage and neuritis are other consequences of alcoholism.

There is little hope for the drinker who expects medicine alone to stop the drinking for him. There are drugs, of which Antabuse is the best known, that will make the patient violently ill if he takes alcohol while the drug is still present in his system.

This sounds like an easy way. It is not. The drug must be given under medical supervision because correct dosage is mandatory. It is also necessary that the patient *take* the drug. The weak link is the chance that the patient will decide that he wants a drink, and the alcoholic, particularly a thirsty alcoholic, can devise all sorts of subterfuges to avoid taking his medicine. If he exerts the necessary will power to keep taking the medicine, he has enough strength of will to stop drinking without the drug.

Alcoholics Anonymous has proved that anyone can give up drinking if he wants to badly enough. After that, whether it is through AA or some other method that the drinker has quit, one rule applies to all: The first drink is too many.

Whether or not alcoholism is a disease has been argued back and forth. Well, it is and it isn't. It is destructive of physical health as well as of emotional and moral well-being, to say nothing of its economic impact. In that sense it is a disease. It may also be counted an emotional disease in the sense that it so often stems from a wish to escape from realities.

It is *not* a disease in the sense that it is something that attacks the patient independent of his behavior. An alcoholic can be an alcoholic only so long as he keeps on drinking of his own volition.

Because calling it a "disease" is sometimes taken by the alcoholic as an excuse, an explanation of why he doesn't stop drinking, it seems to me that there is no point in trying to stretch facts to call it a disease. It is self-indulgence to a harmful degree, and the only cure is to avoid alcohol completely.

A question frequently coming to me, to alcohol clinics, AA chapters and to every doctor, comes from relatives of an alcoholic: "What can I do to help him?"

The answer is that nothing can be done *for* the alcoholic except to help him see himself as he is. Nobody can give up drinking for somebody else. It's as simple as that.

Unfortunately, a great many alcoholics have to come to the point of ruining their lives before they will take the first clear look at themselves. From that point on, they can be helped. But first they must want to be helped.

9

IT'S NOT SKIN DEEP
—THE TRUTH ABOUT ALLERGIES

MAXIM 9 *Learn to be a detective, healthwise, when allergies and many skin problems develop.*

One of my secretaries was a very pretty girl, whose face was perpetually broken out with rashes.

Since a prophet is often without honor in his own country, she ignored me completely. Or perhaps it just didn't occur to her that a physician should be expected to know anything about complexion problems.

I don't know how much she spent on beauty soaps, creams, medications "guaranteed" to give "the beautiful glow of perfect skin," and the rest of the Madison Avenue hyperbole. She went through the whole rigmarole of beauty parlor treatments.

And she still had the rash on her face and was miserable.

One afternoon I just barged into the subject and told her, "See here, you've tried everything imaginable for that skin trouble. Everything but one, that is."

She showed some interest at the suggestion that there might be one thing left to try.

"If you'll do exactly as I say for a month, I'll tell you about the treatment," I said. "But you'll have to agree, absolutely, to follow instructions to the letter."

She promised.

"Just wash your face tonight," I said, "and don't put on a particle of make-up tomorrow morning. Or any time. No medications. No cosmetics of any kind."

"Oh, I couldn't," she said. "This rash is so unsightly. I've got to use enough make-up to cover it."

"You promised," I said.

Reluctantly she agreed to stand by her bargain. Blotchy face and all—without make-up, not even lipstick—she was at work the next day feeling pretty sorry for herself.

But it didn't take a month. In less than a week she could see the difference. The rash continued to clear until it was all gone. On occasion she could use a light touch of lipstick without trouble.

The real trouble was that she had been irritating her skin by the endless collection of things she was using to try to clear it or cover it up.

There's an unhappy ending to the story, so far as I am concerned. She got married and started raising a family, and I lost a good worker. But I'll bet that none of her daughters will go to school heavily made up, the way some do.

Not all skin disorders are allergic in origin. Far from it. And allergies manifest themselves in many ways other than in skin blemishes. They are separate problems, but they overlap to such an extent that we may as well discuss them together. In fact, it is hardly possible to discuss allergy without including skin reactions and equally impossible to talk about skin troubles without considering allergy.

For allergies, some help is possible by medication, but if you hope to acquire protection against future attacks, one fact is absolutely necessary: *You must find out what food or material is causing the attacks.* This requires a good deal of medical detective work on the part of both patient and doctor. More about this later.

Sometimes the disease is readily apparent in skin ailments. Other times it, too, must be the subject of detective work. Keep-

ing in mind the interconnection of the two subjects, let's turn
now to the skin.

THINK OF SKIN AS AN ORGAN

If you are to take care of any organ of the body intelligently
and effectively, and to know how to recognize signs of illness and
how to avoid illnesses, you have to understand the rudiments of
how the organ works.

This is true of the skin, for the skin *is* an organ, the largest of
the body—extending from crown to toes.

Learn to think of it as more than a passive covering for the
body. It is a protective covering, to be sure, but it is much more
than that, and it is scarcely passive.

Through its sweat glands, it provides water for evaporation,
thus cooling the body.

It is active in the formation of antibodies for protection against
germs.

It embraces a network of nerve endings—the sense of touch.

It excretes, along with water, some minerals.

It exudes oils (called sebum) for its protection.

It produces Vitamin D through action of sunlight.

Is the skin an organ? It certainly is, and a most complex one.

The skin includes the nails and the hair. Both are subject to
certain skin afflictions. Infections can cause loss of hair; fungus
infections are the most prevalent cause of nail trouble, with the
exception of brittleness, which I'll mention later.

But the skin has remarkable tolerance and its own ways of
protecting itself. Under pressure, it forms a callus. Or if irritation
or pressure is rapid and severe, it creates a blister as emergency
protection.

Skins, of course, vary greatly in texture. Some are coarse, some
smooth. Blonds and redheads are more vulnerable to sunburn
than are brunettes. Some persons are vulnerable to athlete's foot,
for example—and others are not. Some tolerate irritants such as
oil or household chemicals. Some do not. The same variations
occur in hair and nails.

The skin is a useful barometer of health—the pink skin of glowing health, the pallor of anemia, dryness with thyroid deficiency, duskiness with circulatory disorders. It may also reveal our emotional state—the blush of embarrassment, or—well, from here on, suppose we take, one by one, a number of the most frequent complaints concerning the skin.

Excessive perspiration This is usually seen in the nervous or sensitive person, but it isn't always easy to convince a patient. Many a doctor has encountered the patient who says tensely, "But doctor, I'm *not* upset about anything. There's nothing worrying me. I assure you of that. All I want is something to slow down the amount of perspiration because it isn't normal. Other people don't sweat this much!"

He's not tense? The tension is apparent in every word he says, but *he* doesn't think he is, because that's the way he always is!

Antiperspirants can help to a considerable degree, but not when the heavy perspiration is generalized, but most annoying in the palms, armpits and feet.

Sedation may help. The gradual growth of self-confidence almost always does. The goal is to get the patient to relax.

(One exception to this is "night sweats," which may be a sign of infection, particularly some unrecognized infection which has developed. Tuberculosis, which creeps up with so little warning, is one of these.)

Unpleasant odor serves only to make the nervous patient that much more nervous. It often helps, however, to explain that sweat itself has no odor. The odor comes from bacterial activity on the surface as well as from an oily secretion from specialized (apocrine) glands. These are concentrated in armpits and genital areas.

Clearly we are not all the same in the amount or type of bacteria we carry on our skins. Naturally, cleanliness is a necessity, but some folks have more of a problem than others, for reasons not well understood. Dusting the armpits with ordinary baking soda has helped some. Medicated soaps may be worth a try in some cases.

Psoriasis This accounts for about 5 percent of all skin disorders. It remains a mystery. Neither the cause nor any specific cure is known. There appears to be a strong hereditary factor, but that does not explain all of it by any means.

A multitude of treatments exist, and all fail in some cases. It is perhaps true that all succeed in some cases, too!

About 30 percent of cases tend to recover spontaneously, so there isn't too much question but that some remedies have been credited with cases that were going to clear up anyway.

Psoriasis waxes and wanes in intensity, sometimes with the seasons, usually being less troublesome in summer. For all its appearance, it isn't catching and is not dangerous.

The multiplicity of remedies is evidence of its stubbornness, and patients quite often change doctors and treatments too quickly for any to do much good. It is better to remain with a single doctor, and let him try different treatments as seems advisable. Hoping that some other doctor will happen onto the right treatment is pretty much like leaving the whole thing to luck.

There is no known way to avoid psoriasis. It is one of those things.

Acne This bane of the teen-ager is another matter. Something *can* be done about it, and it can do more positive harm than the unsightly but innocuous psoriasis.

With adolescence the glandular activity of the body is changing, for the body is undergoing the transition from childhood to adulthood. The sebaceous glands of the skin are awakening to activity. These are the countless little glands which emit oily material.

The condition called acne occurs when some of the glands become plugged by this otherwise useful material. Blackheads often form, the black head being an oily material that turns dark on exposure to the air. That is why, when a blackhead is expelled, the top is black and the rest a whitish or creamy color.

The little gland swells, becomes inflamed, and even may become infected. This last possibility is responsible for most of the pitting and scarring.

Squeezing out the blackheads with the fingernails should *not* be attempted. Too often the squeezing damages the skin around it. Using a needle is even worse. At the drugstore you can get blackhead expressors (simple little metal gadgets), which will help press out the blackheads with minimum damage.

Always keep in mind the cause: The heavy flow of pasty, oily material, and the fact that it sometimes clogs the gland.

Hence, cleanliness is important. Here is some advice for the acne-beset teen-ager: Wash frequently, a number of times a day. Do some gentle scrubbing with a soft facial brush. Do not use a stiff brush. Don't scrub so hard that the skin is reddened. What you are trying to do is loosen and brush away some of the oily substance, without scratching the skin. For even a tiny scratch is a potential gateway for infection. After the scrubbing, rinse copiously. Lots of fresh water will wash away bits of the loosened material.

Emotions seem to play a big role. The more the youngster frets about the acne, the worse it becomes. If you can get across the idea that this is a temporary problem, and that it can be eased by handling it correctly, you usually have the battle half won. It will take time, but visible progress will cut the vicious cycle of acne-nerves-more acne.

Diet is a factor. Sea foods, chocolate, nuts, cola drinks are the most frequent offenders in aggravating (although they cannot be said to cause) acne. It is best to eliminate all of them and to stick to a diet that is low in fat.

Lotions may be used to soften or dissolve the thin layer of material which is clogging a gland, letting the rest work its way out. Lotions containing sulphur will help, and tend to reduce the amount of oily secretion. In cases that have become severely infected, antibiotics may be required for a time. Vitamin A has been helpful in some instances, although this is not true for all.

And in a few years the trouble almost always comes to an end, but "a few years" to a teen-ager sounds like centuries.

A youngster fretting about acne needs a lot of reassurance, needs to have something to do to help the condition, and needs to see some progress.

Dermatitis This is a very general term—inflammation of the skin. We'll talk later about the heavier, localized infections, such as boils. They could, in a sense, be called a "dermatitis," but "infection" better describes them.

There are scores of varieties of dermatitis. I believe it to be entirely pointless to try to list even part of them, much less suggest treatments. An atopic or an allergic dermatitis would not be aided at all (might indeed be aggravated) by a treatment specified for, let's say, ringworm. Sunburn (a form of dermatitis) requires quite different treatment than dermatitis rhus, which is a handsome name for poison ivy or poison oak.

It may sound as though I'm not going to give you any handy home treatments for dermatitis. That's right. I'm not.

Instead, I'm going to beg you not to fool around with salves, lotions or home remedies for skin trouble.

You'll be vastly better off by having either your doctor or a skin specialist see your case before you have done anything to it.

I have yet to talk to a dermatologist who hasn't bemoaned this very point. Many skin ailments are not easily diagnosed except by someone who has studied care of the skin in great detail.

Time after time patients finally arrive at the doctor's office only after weeks or months of trying this or that salve, lotion or ointment that somebody recommended.

By that time, the "treatments" have so additionally inflamed the skin that, until the medicine-instigated irritation has been allowed to subside, it is often impossible to determine what the original trouble was.

Meanwhile the patient becomes angry, wondering why the doctor doesn't do something to cure him. And the doctor can't, until he can see what the basic trouble may be.

Warts and moles   Warts are a thickening of the outer layer of skin, and with a few exceptions aren't worthy of concern. The cause is a virus, probably more than one kind of virus.

The wart cures practiced by Tom Sawyer and Huckleberry Finn probably are as adequate as any. Frankly, I forget just what mumbo jumbo those famous boys used. Seems to me it involved a chicken killed and buried under a full moon, with some incantations by Huck.

For economy's sake, better use some of the other old favorites, such as putting half of a fresh-cut potato or onion over the wart, standing on one foot and facing west.

Vociferous as I am against most old granny potions and notions, this is the exception, because these silly wart cures seem to work a good deal of the time. Maybe the real reason is that warts, like colds, run their course in due time anyway.

As to tying a thread around a wart until it falls off— well, I have intellectual reservations against anything that smacks of cutting off the circulation, but I don't have any concrete evidence of anyone being harmed by the thread cure. Perhaps it is because I don't know of anyone who ever continued this treatment longer than the span of a small boy's interest, which isn't very long.

In instances in which it really seems imperative to do something about warts, there are various treatments usually involving salicylic acid. Or cauterization is effective, and in some cases, as in plantar warts, ultrasound has been used. X ray, too.

When a crop of warts appears, it has often been noted that removal of a few of them is followed by disappearance of the rest. One theory is that tampering with one wart may instigate a defense mechanism that causes others to disappear. I personally like the "shiny new quarter cure." Rub it on each wart. Presto! The warts often disappear. I have seen it work!

Plantar warts appear on the plantar, or sole, portion of the foot, a most annoying and painful place for warts. They have a nasty habit of recurring, conceivably because the moist warmth of the foot encourages them.

Sometimes it is sufficient for the doctor to pare them off, for comfort. If new ones persist, some of the more sophisticated treatments are advised. The patient meanwhile should take precautions against passing the plantar wart virus on to others in the family. He should not walk barefoot around the house but should wear slippers or clogs.

Moles are more common than warts. It is said that nobody is without at least a tiny mole somewhere. Yet the cause is unknown. Certain skin pigments gather, and that is that. They may be of varying shades of brown or blue-black. Some are red, since they contain blood vessels. Some moles are hairy, some not. (*Never* pull a hair from a mole. If the hair annoys you, snip it off with scissors.)

Sometimes we are born with moles. Sometimes moles appear later. In fact, it is known that moles tend to appear with the passage of time. Generally speaking, moles are not harmful, but may be cosmetically disfiguring, in which case they can be removed readily by a dermatologist or a plastic surgeon.

Any change in size, color or texture of a mole, or any tendency of a mole to bleed, warrants removal, because these changes sometimes precede cancer. So long as you are watchful, and act promptly in case of any change, you have no cause for worry. Most moles never cause any trouble. If one is so located as to be irritated by clothing—brassière, belt, strap, garter, collar or whatever—have it removed for safety. But don't, unless for the sake of appearance, fuss about removal of a mole unless you have noted some change, or it is being constantly irritated.

As for various birthmarks, "port wine" marks, or hemangiomas (a proliferation of small blood vessels) or other such marks— nearly all can be successfully removed surgically. Some are disposed of by freezing with Dry Ice. Many times experts suggest waiting for a time to see whether a mark will diminish or disappear by itself.

There are no home remedies of any sort, but medical (or surgical) treatment is highly effective, so don't be unduly upset about a birthmark on a baby. And please help eliminate the plethora of old wives' tales about babies being marked because their mothers ate strawberries, or were frightened by something or did or didn't do something or other. These folklore fables are long-lived, but there is nothing to them.

Sebaceous cysts   It is not unusual for a sebaceous (oil) gland to become encysted. That is, the duct from it becomes completely closed. This is apart from the temporary clogging as in acne. A cyst implies permanent closure.

Yet the gland, by its nature, continues to produce the material it is intended to provide. The material cannot escape, so the gland swells. This is *not* a malignant, or cancerous, condition. It can, however, be painful sometimes. If they cause no trouble, these cysts can be left alone. If they hurt or become infected, then they should have attention—and the right kind of attention.

The habit of having such a thing lanced, or opened with a sharp instrument, is an old one but outdated for most purposes. Opening a cyst will afford quick relief by relieving the pressure but will effect no permanent cure. The cyst will seal itself again, and the pressure will mount again.

The way to get rid of a cyst permanently is to have the entire cyst (that is, the entire gland) removed. Often this is a simple office procedure. However, there are times when the cyst lies somewhat deeper and may require very careful handling to avoid deranging muscles or other tissues. Two or three days or so in the hospital may be required, in some cases. Don't be surprised if this is the case, even though the cyst may, on the surface, seem to be a very small one. Office surgery usually; brief hospital care sometimes.

Growths and skin cancer   Skin cancer is one of the readily detectable types of cancer. For that reason it is one of the most curable of cancers. Remove it early, and success is probable. With the exception of skin cancers that people do not report to their doctors, such cancers are curable in ninety-odd percent of all cases. Nearly all can be removed successfully.

In fact, in many instances it is a misnomer to call some of these things cancer. They are neoplastic areas—new growth of tissue where there should be no growth. They are potentially cancerous, or precancerous, and removing them before they actually become malignant is simpler than it is if we wait until biopsies show that actual cancer is present.

Such growths, usually as we get along in years, often appear on the forehead, bridge of the nose, temples. Some horny growths at times appear on the ears. So just tell your doctor as soon as you notice such a growth. Or if something resembling a sore appears and does not heal within a couple of weeks.

Skin cancer is more prevalent among people who are out in the sun a great deal.

Infections   Infectious organisms are all around us, particularly the staphylococcus germ. The skin does a very good job of keeping them out. The little space around a hair, if in some way damaged slightly, is a favored place for the entry of such germs.

This invasion, and the multiplication of germs, is a boil, or furuncle. A number of them, close together and forming a large mass, is a carbuncle.

In some areas a boil can be, as the expression goes, "sore as a boil." Other boils may not be nearly so sensitive. The explanation lies in the tissue in which the boil forms. In the ear, for example, little expansion of the tissues is possible, so pressure in the boil builds up quickly, and pain is severe. In softer areas, the tissues are subjected to less pressure because they can stretch.

Treatment of a boil? You may want your doctor to take care of it if it becomes too painful. If you attempt to take care of it yourself, remember this cardinal rule: The area around it must be kept antiseptically clean. The boil should be covered with a simple dressing.

Your goal is to prevent matter in the boil from escaping to spread to the roots of other hairs and start more boils. When one has a "crop of boils," the reason is *not* that the infection is "in the blood." Boils develop from the outside, not from the inside.

Keep the surface clean!

Excess hair It is rarely a health problem, but it certainly is a problem that excites a vast number of inquiries. A few typical questions are these:

> What can I do about dark hair that has started coming on my upper lip? What causes this? Is it gland trouble?

This from a mother:

> My daughter is 15. She had medicine for a bad attack of the flu a year ago. Now she is getting this dark growth of hair. Could the medicine cause that?

From a daughter:

> My girl friends shave their legs but my mother won't let me because she says it will make the hair heavier. What can I do? I want to look nice.

Glandular disorders occasionally cause heavy growth of hair, but "occasionally" is all I mean. Such disorders (tumors of the ovary, perhaps, or adrenal glands) are not common.

Most "excessive" hair isn't excessive at all, from the standpoint of normal health. It is excessive only to the degree that we don't want it.

Inherited racial characteristics are the most important controlling factor. The hair of the light-skinned person often is light, too, and scarcely visible. So the brunettes are usually the ones who complain.

Precious few medications cause or encourage growth of hair, and none of those commonly used do. If they could, they would soon enough be used to restore hair to bald heads—and nobody has found a way to do that. (In some instances scalp dermatitis may be the cause of baldness. If the dermatitis is treated and halted in time, it can prevent the baldness. But most baldness is, like excessive hair, a matter of heredity and not controllable.)

The answer to the question quoted above is doubtless a simple one: The medicine had nothing to do with it. The appearance of hair was quite natural.

The remedies for unwanted hair are few but effective, and it is fruitless to search hopefully for something that will change your inborn characteristics.

Bleaching makes hairs less noticeable.

Plucking them is temporary in effect. They ordinarily grow in again.

Depilatories—chemicals which dissolve the hairs—are used by many. But they, too, are of temporary effect. The hairs grow back and can be dissolved away again. (Some sensitive skins are irritated by these products, in which case some other method will have to be used. For most people they are effective and satisfactory.)

Shaving does *not* make hair grow back in heavier, coarser, darker or faster. This is a misconception shared by both sexes. Adolescent boys start shaving the first fuzz in the hope of growing a heavier beard. Mothers of adolescent girls tell their daughters not to shave their legs because they fear it will make the hair heavier. Both are mistaken. Women from 16 to 60-odd can shave their legs without encouraging any increased growth. Boys can shave twice a day throughout their teens but will still have exactly the same beard that Nature intended. If you doubt it, what about some of the religious or other groups which raise bushy black beards and never shave?

Finally, the one permanent way of removing unwanted hair is to have it removed by electrolysis, which destroys the roots. This has to be done one hair at a time, so it is painstaking. If permanent removal isn't worth that, then settle for one of the other methods.

Pruritus (another name for itching)   At the beginning of this chapter we remarked that the skin contains the ends of sensory nerves. Any subtle irritation can cause itching.

It may be some chemical irritant. Or mild infection. Or parasites. A mosquito bite itches, too.

It may be of allergic origin, something you touched or ate, or something in the air. More of that in the allergy section.

It may be that the skin has become too dry.

Or some systemic disease, such as jaundice, leukemia, diabetes, a blood disorder and so forth, can have itching as a symptom.

And it may be psychological, or "psychosomatic" if you like. Neurodermatitis is a localized itching, affecting some patch of skin, without any external stimulus that we can find. Nerves can make you itch.

Pruritus, pronounced prue-*right*-uss, is a mighty prevalent trouble.

Here, as in some of the other skin conditions, your detective work is important. Especially important here. When do you itch? Where? I suggest that you abstain from trying to make a diagnosis yourself. But observe all the evidence you can. Be a good witness, but don't try to be prosecutor and judge besides. This involves a principle (I think it's a principle) that extends to things wholly beyond the realm of medicine. If you are a witness, confine yourself to testifying to the facts. If you are a prosecutor, try to draw out the pertinent facts on one side. If a defense attorney, the facts on the other side. If a judge, or a juror, try to weigh the facts on both sides and reach a decision.

In medicine, be a perfect witness as a patient. As a doctor, try to be the most dispassionate judge or juror.

This is a thought to which I allude elsewhere in this tome, but the concept is a valid, useful one. As in life we have found that trying to be both witness and juror, both prosecutor and judge, leads to inherent error; we have also found that you can't be both doctor and patient at the same time.

Or to boil it down to cases, or better yet to the present case, don't itch and then go to the doctor and say, "I itch. I have pruritus. It's an allergy." Just tell the doctor that you itch. And where. And under what circumstances. Place on his shoulders the responsibility of deciding whether it is an allergy or something else.

A couple of very common causes of pru . . . well, itching, merit special comment. One is from overdryness, from overbathing, especially in winter, and very frequent among older people. Their skins, too oily at 17, are too dry at 70. Too much soap and water at the latter age removes the now-scarce oils. Or the house is kept quite warm and not very humid; that dries out the skin. Result? Itch. Remedy? Use humidifiers. Wash enough to keep clean but not enough to remove oils. Use bath oils or creams after the bath.

Another very common complaint is "detergent hands." Detergents, by their very nature, are designed to remove greasy residues. That's one of the big reasons why detergents have become so useful as cleaning compounds.

Most of us can use detergents for household cleaning, especially dishes, without any consequences. But some of us, and believe me, I've seen hundreds and had letters from thousands, have trouble. Thousands, out of millions of people, is a rather small proportion, but that is no consolation for the sufferers.

Is it allergy? Perhaps, at times. But it may also be the simpler explanation that removal of oils from the hands irritates them.

Seldom, apparently, does this business of "detergent hands" come on suddenly. Women put up with the itching at first. They manage to stand it for a time after the hands become red and the skin cracks. When they can't bear to tackle another sinkful of dishes, they at last appeal to their doctors, or to me.

By then it is too late to expect some emollient to restore the skin so it can at once stand the irritation. The skin will need time to recover. Creams containing lanolin or the like will help. Keep the hands out of water. Use rubber gloves, and if they, too, irritate (which may be the case) get cotton-lined ones, or even wear cotton gloves inside the rubber.

You may in time be able to take some liberties with detergents again. Next time start protecting your skin early instead of late. Apply this same thought to any skin irritation. The skin does not as a rule break down easily. When it does, it must have time to rebuild.

Another quite prevalent form of itching is neurodermatitis (localized itching partly and sometimes wholly due to psychological causes). It tends to come and go, may or may not move from place to place. It often occurs during or following periods of stress, anger, anxiety, frustration and annoyance.

By hard experience, dermatologists soon come to recognize these cases of "psychological itch," and in the same way they have come to know that many patients resent being told the cause, or refuse to accept it. If often takes a lot of subtle and laborious coaxing before the patient is ready to go along with some really effective treatment. I hope my readers will not be so reluctant.

One of the most vivid examples of this to come to my attention was that of a man who suffered unbearably from rectal itching, or pruritus ani, which is a pretty common affliction.

(Of course the first step is to make sure that no physical cause is at work—no hemorrhoids, crypts, fissures. Some care should be taken to determine whether a food allergy is involved.

With these ruled out, very often the answer is extreme cleanliness—washing with soap and water to be sure that no tiny particles of matter remain to irritate. And after that, thorough drying, and sometimes the placing of a tiny wad of cotton, to absorb all moisture.)

This man had gone through all of that and tried all manner of salves, suppositories and medications. No success. In desperation he finally agreed to see a psychiatrist. It took six visits, he told me. And his itching stopped.

Dandruff Not much to say about this, really, except that amazingly few people seem to know what it is. It is a scalp disorder from microorganisms of the yeast or fungus family, causing scaling, or flaking, itch, loss of hair. Contributing factors include conditions of heat, humidity, dust, hormone balance. Mild infection may set in.

Careful shampooing is essential. If this alone does not succeed, medicated shampoos are available to reduce scaling, promote drying and attack the fungus or yeast.

Aging skin   Decreases in both perspiration and oil production as we grow older make the skin drier and contribute to itching. Avoidance of overwashing, use of lanolin creams, humidifying the house, especially in winter, are the best answers.

Wrinkling does not, in my experience, respond to any notable degree to any sort of medication. It is due to loss of weight and to decreased elasticity of the underlying supporting tissues.

Within reasonable limits, face lifting is successful, but good judgment is required. Premature sagging (under the eyes, for example) can be corrected by plastic surgery, but this sort of procedure should be limited to making the face look as young as one really is—not younger.

In scarred skin cases, dermatologists and plastic surgeons can help greatly by "skin planing," which is a process of removing the outer portions of the skin with high-speed rotary brushes or other methods. Be guided by professional counsel as to whether any particular case will benefit. It has its limitations.

Brittle nails   An annoyance, often, rather than a true health problem, but a very frequent complaint. Women like to grow long, carefully shaped nails. Breaking them is bound to be more frequent.

Hard manual work is known to strengthen and toughen nails —but how this can be accomplished while still keeping long nails, I don't know. It's a choice people must make for themselves.

Excessively brittle nails can reflect some protein deficiency, which explains the popularity of taking plain gelatin. Gelatin is an incomplete form of protein. It may sometimes help the nails. Since I see no harm in taking it, I have no objection to anyone trying it, but it certainly cannot produce results until enough time has passed for nails to grow out. The strength is established as the nail is forming in the nail bed. I frankly doubt that gelatin will do any better than a diet just ordinarily high in protein foods.

How to Identify Allergies

I have written very often about allergy.

Why? Because it is so often overlooked as a cause of various ills. And because it is so common.

At least 70 percent of us have at least minor allergies. It is possible, I suppose, that nearly all of us might be found to be allergic to something, if we hunted long enough.

What is allergy? It is hypersensitivity, extreme sensitivity, to some substance that does not provoke any visible response in a normal individual.

You may be quite normal as regards one substance yet react intensely to a whiff or a taste or the touch of something else. One man's food is another's poison—such useful and wholesome products as wool, wheat, eggs, milk, oats are often causes of childhood allergies.

Pity the mother of twins, one of whom proved to be allergic to wheat and the other to oats. She had to prepare one type of cereal for one, a different cereal for the other, and had to keep straight in her mind which twin was which, and which twin had which allergy. Yes, it really happened.

Minor allergies may manifest themselves in occasional sneezes, occasional hives, occasional diarrhea, itching, weepy eyes, runny noses. A lot of childhood "colds," especially if they hang on, can be allergic reactions rather than virus infections. The signs are much the same: drippy nose, mild cough, perhaps wheezing.

Some allergies tend to fade later on, particularly if they are recognized early and a child is protected from the things which bother him. He then has time to develop some tolerance.

Eczema in babies is due to allergy about 75 percent of the time, usually a food allergy. Usually there will be a history of minor allergies in the parents—sometimes minor enough so that the parents themselves haven't thought much about it.

I've come across a good variety of such cases, not to mention the mysterious rashes that were traced to a sensitivity to a wool blanket or baby bonnet, or to feathers in a pillow. Feathers are another frequent offender.

We feed babies so carefully! We try to start them at the right time on the foods that are good for them, and unless we are alert, we forget that some of these perfectly healthful foods will, at times, touch off allergic responses.

If we forget that, we may have a most baffling time, trying to figure out what ails a little one. But we should keep that thought strongly fixed in mind, for since we usually introduce one new food at a time to a baby, we are able to spot, or at least suspect, a food allergy right from the start.

Another complication is that allergic responses may take quite different forms: rashes and eczema, or the false cold, or asthmatic wheezing, or giant hives or swelling. I know one little fellow, at first thought to be uncommonly stubborn, who from babyhood was suspicious of just about every new food offered to him. Given a spoonful of spinach, he would blow it all over his tray, not to mention his mother.

It turned out that he was allergic to green vegetables and had the good sense not to let anyone feed them to him. This aspect of his allergy ultimately disappeared, but he had many others. Egg bothered him greatly, and several years later I saw his lips and mouth swell grotesquely, within minutes of his innocently eating part of a cookie which contained egg.

So sometimes the reaction is immediate, sometimes somewhat delayed, sometimes this, sometimes that as a symptom; some really tricky detective work may be needed.

One Big Help—A Food Diary

Where food allergy is suspected, a food diary is a most useful thing—a record, meal by meal, and between meals, of everything eaten.

For the first few days and perhaps for several weeks, it may seem to be a jumble. But along with the food record, there should be a notation of everything that seems to be an allergic reaction, and its duration. (It is helpful to enter these notes in a different colored ink.)

Then, as one skims back over the food diary, things gradually begin to fit into a pattern. A certain food has a way of appearing just before each attack.

Don't think it's easy. It's not. But hit-or-miss guesswork is generally futile.

With an older child or an adult, allergists often use another approach—limiting the patient to an extremely simple diet consisting of a few foods which infrequently cause trouble. After a period of this, assuming that allergic attacks have subsided, other foods are added, one at a time and at intervals of a few days. When trouble starts again, one offending food has been exposed by the detective work.

The patient rarely needs much persuasion to leave such foods alone, even though they may, at times, be things of which he is extremely fond.

The one way of avoiding trouble is to avoid the cause. Although antihistamine drugs can be helpful in some types of allergy, usually nasal allergies, they are of little use with food sensitivities.

USE OF THE ANTIHISTAMINES

Since we've mentioned antihistaminic medications, this is a good time to outline briefly the way allergies behave. We understand it only within limits. Certain substances cause the release, from the body's tissues, of a material called histamine. Histamine has its uses. In some conditions it becomes a drug valued as a diagnostic tool, as well for treatment.

But the sudden release of histamine seems to play irritable havoc. Hence, the distress is alleviated by antihistaminic drugs, which suppress the activity of the histamine.

When the antihistamines first became available they were seized upon as a "cold cure." (This was strongly opposed by the discoverer of the first such drug, and the people associated with him, but they were shouted down for a time by the "cold cure" faction.)

The real significance, of course, was the prevalence of allergic rhinitis, or allergy-producing cold symptoms. These cases were helped by antihistamines. True colds are not.

Useful as these drugs are, they cannot be considered a cure. They relieve the symptoms. They do not change the basic condition. (In many individuals, they may cause drowsiness, and it is well to avoid them if you are going to be driving an automobile.)

The steroid hormones (the cortisone family) also are powerfully effective in suppressing symptoms. They, even more, must be used with caution, because of side effects which can become truly dangerous. They are extremely valuable in emergencies.

Most perilous of all allergens are drugs. Pollen, foods, dust and other everyday materials, annoying as they may be, represent little threat to life. Drugs may be quite another matter.

Even the old reliable aspirin can be dangerous, sometimes even deadly, to someone highly hypersensitive to it. One of the best known of such drug sensitivities is that of penicillin. This is one of several reasons why this fine antibiotic must not be employed indiscriminately.

First use of such a drug will not carry the risk. Only after the patient has become "sensitized" by being exposed to the drug, one or perhaps many times, does the danger develop. But people so sensitized have been dangerously affected. On some occasions, the tissues of their air passages have swollen so severely that only prompt treatment prevented their dying from lack of oxygen.

It is in emergencies such as these that adrenalin or the steroids are invaluable.

But enough of these near-tragic occurrences. Let's get back to the control of allergies in our everyday lives.

THAT AUTUMN SCAMP, HAY FEVER

Hay fever, hypersensitivity to pollen, too often is attributed solely to pollen from ragweed in the fall. Ragweed is, indeed, the great offender, but a whole squad of other weeds, trees and grasses do their part of the dirty work.

Earlier in the growing season, "rose fever" brings on similar complaints, although grasses and other plants, rather than roses, do the mischief. It is not unusual to encounter, at times, someone who "gets a cold" from mowing the lawn or breaks out in a rash from picking a bunch of flowers or even brushing against some shrubbery.

In a good many instances, the result can be a headache—the "histamine headache" being an identified entity.

Since ragweed and other pollens can be carried for miles by the wind (and even detected far out at sea), it isn't easy to escape it. Some spots in the United States, along the Canadian border, are far enough north for the pollen count to be very low. Still, while most of us can't trot off on vacation when the pollen season arrives, we can stay in town rather than in the country. The less pollen the better.

If we have other known allergies, we can be extra-cautious. Most people with any marked degree of allergy are sensitive to a number of allergens, not to just one—and allergenic response tends to be additive. One type of attack contributes to another, in the sense that the patient's total tolerance is that much more exhausted.

Some (not all) sufferers find that air conditioning brings relief, and they spend time in theaters, department stores or other air-conditioned buildings, and sometimes have air conditioning at home, or devices which filter pollen and dust from the air in a room.

But the most successful approach of all is desensitization—treatment with minute quantities of the allergens far in advance of the season, with gradual increase in amount to build up a tolerance.

Some begin this in winter. Others, and wisely, carry on such desensitization treatment the year round. There are few who do not benefit from it. The majority achieve very great relief. They may, although this is not always so, have to keep up the treatments indefinitely. People do get over hay fever, but infrequently.

Effective treatment is of value more than just for the sake of the relief it affords in the hay-fever season. A substantial number of hay-fever sufferers eventually develop asthma, which in turn incites a variety of lung disorders and can overwork the heart.

ALL WHEEZES ARE NOT ASTHMA

All wheezy breathing is not asthma. Emphysema, chronic bronchitis, bronchial tumors, congestive heart disease—these are other possibilities.

We can say, however, that most wheezers have asthma, a spasmodic constriction of the bronchial tubes making it difficult to breathe. Allergies quite unrelated to pollen or hay fever may be responsible.

The list of possibilities is hopelessly long: animal danders, feathers of a pillow or a parrot, house dust, foods, plants, fabrics, weather changes (temperature as well as humidity). Endless. Some common infection can set off an asthma attack, because it is quite possible for a person to be hypersensitive to bacteria.

If children can be freed of asthma by the time they are 10 to 12 years old, it is an excellent portent. They may remain free of it, or at least be able to control the condition by being careful.

But bringing this about usually implies careful treatment in the early years, for asthma does not show any tendency to get better spontaneously. It is quite the opposite. It grows worse.

Every effort should be made to pin down the causes of asthma. From 10 to 20 percent of asthma cases defy treatment; the rest yield to removal of allergens, desensitization, drugs to relax and decongest the bronchial system and make breathing easier.

And not the least factor is emotional or psychological. Some authorities who have studied asthma intensively work on the assumption that allergy and emotional tension will be present in every case of asthma. This is not hard to believe, when you have struggled with a good many cases.

This is not to say that emotional upsets *cause* asthma, but they most decidedly play a part in triggering an attack. And the asthma itself, with difficult breathing and a sense of impending suffocation, reinforces the whole unhappy sequence.

SOME MORE DETECTIVE WORK

Another large and separate category is contact dermatitis—skin irritation from touching something. This may or may not be strictly allergic in origin. That, however, is a bit academic. If contact with something bothers your skin, find out what it is.

This sounds simple. Yet often it is just as brain-teasing as unmasking a food allergen. Metals (especially nickel), soaps, cosmetics, oils, detergents, ink, plastics, paint, carbon paper, dyes, perfumes are a few examples.

When the sensitivity is to the rubber in a girdle (as has happened) the pattern of the skin irritation is an obvious enough clue. Or when, as also happened, a surgeon turned out to be sensitive to a certain kind of surgical gloves.

But when the irritation is on the fingers or only part of the hands, it may be extremely hard to guess which of the scores or hundreds of things touched may be the culprit. The exact shape and extent of the skin rash may be a clue if you figure it out carefully enough. You hold a broom one way, a telephone another, a door key in still another. The paint on a broom handle was the answer in one case, something in the plastic of the phone in another, the metal of a frequently used key in still another. (It was a tough one when irritation on a man's finger tips seemed to have no answer—until his allergist noticed the patient's habit of jingling coins in his pocket. Silver and copper didn't bother him, but nickel did!)

Jewelry, and perhaps more particularly costume jewelry, sometimes irritates. A clear lacquer has been successfully used many times to prevent direct contact of metal and skin, so that favorite earrings or necklaces needn't be abandoned.

And that's a small outline of a very big topic.

A FEW FINAL REMARKS

I have touched rather fleetingly on direct testing for allergies—skin tests or patch tests. These are useful, much-used, but sometimes misleading tests.

Allergists have available extracts of a large number of frequently encountered allergens, but it would be utterly impossible to check all of them.

Yes, these sensitivity tests are a great help in tracking allergens,

but they are (as your allergist will doubtless warn you) sometimes guilty of giving false positives, or of giving a positive indication when the patient's sensitivity may not be especially great.

House dust, feathers, any of the common items may be pretty
well eliminated from suspicion with such tests, but there is no
guarantee that the really strong offenders necessarily will be
included in the tests. So keep your detecting wits about you, and
do not fall into the optimistic error of expecting that a course of
skin tests and some desensitization shots will clear up everything
for you. That's oversimplifying a very difficult situation.

We should add a word about a problem that is looming as more
important than we once thought: insect stings, particularly of
the bee-wasp-hornet group. Once a person has become sensitized
by a prior sting or stings (not everybody will, naturally, but some
may), reaction to subsequent stings can be violent indeed. I
thoroughly credit reports that such insect bites cause more deaths
than snakebites.

Desensitization against this danger is available, if you have
reason to believe you have become sensitized.

A closing suggestion: Persons known to have a high degree of
allergy should carry a warning with them, as diabetics or people
with serious heart conditions do, in case of emergency. Since
tetanus antitoxin is often used in first-aid treatment of burns or
wounds, and this is ordinarily a horse serum product, anyone
sensitive to horse serum will avoid both trouble and danger by
carrying such a warning. So many individuals have become sensitized to penicillin and other drugs or materials, that a warning
of this can be lifesaving.

10

ARE YOU OUT OF JOINT?

MAXIM 10 *A few logical precautions will save an immense amount of trouble—and worry—concerning the joints and muscles. A useful tip: Remember that every twinge and every pain isn't necessarily arthritis.*

This complicated body of ours is made up skeletally of nearly 200 bones and about 500 muscles.

For nearly every bone there is a joint. True, in a few instances several bones fuse together and become essentially one. The skull is an example of this.

But other areas are exceedingly complex. A wrist and hand have 27 bones, and an equivalent number of bearing surfaces or joints. The wrist, since it must turn in every direction, is a marvelous and complicated example of Nature's engineering.

For that matter, every joint is a beautifully efficient device. The joining bones are held together—and also cushioned—by cartilage and ligaments. A band of ligaments encases the joint; this is called the joint capsule. Inside it, a thin membrane retains a fluid (synovial fluid) which is the lubricant for the joint.

Movement, of course, is governed by the muscles—or rather pairs of muscles or pairs of groups of muscles. With the finger, one set of muscles crooks or flexes the finger. Another group, working in opposition, straightens or extends the finger. And so for other joints, one set pulls one way, another set pulls oppositely. This is an oversimplified way of putting it. Just crook your finger forward, and notice the way certain of the joints operate independently. Or you can hold the finger straight yet bend it forward at the big knuckle. Other groups of muscles draw it from side to side.

Some joints are relatively insecure and thus subject to dislocation, but this is a matter of necessity. The shoulder has to move in all directions and move to a considerable degree, too. Try it—your arm up, down, forward, back, straight out or across in front of you. You can hunch your shoulders forward, or up or hold them back. Pretty wonderful mechanism, isn't it? And besides all this the shoulder absorbs a great deal of punishment: football, carrying heavy burdens, lifting, twisting, pushing. The wonder is that we have so little trouble with our shoulders, not that we have so much.

Other joints, as hip, knee and ankle, must be under continued stress. They have to carry our weight. They are subject to impact from all directions.

A "baseball finger" is a sore, swollen joint, irritated when a ball hits the end of the finger. A "tennis elbow" rebels because it has been subjected to too much stress, and it becomes sore.

In certain of the joints strong tendons are in use. The "hamstring" muscles in back of the knee, which you can readily feel, and the "Achilles tendon" at the heel are easily identified tendons. Little fluid-filled sacs, called bursae, are provided for them to ride over smoothly. When a bursa becomes inflamed from a blow, or too much continued pressure, or any other cause, we have bursitis.

There was a famous and unhappy case in which a noted politician got bursitis in his shoulder in the midst of a campaign, and it played hob with his hand-shaking. "Housemaid's knee" is a classic example, the bursae of the kneecaps protesting prolonged pressure.

"Tennis elbow" is bursitis. So is "chauffeur's elbow," the pressure in that case coming from resting the arm too often on the hard edge of a car window.

The shoulder is the likeliest place for bursitis. If the bursa is becoming irritated, a bump or blow, or the strain of washing walls or painting can set off an attack.

WHAT TO DO ABOUT IT

In severe cases, even narcotics may be needed to control the pain for a short time. Hot, wet compresses help. Injections of hydrocortisone may give instantaneous relief, although not always. X ray and ultrasound therapy may be used.

And—it may sound silly to say this—the affected part should be rested. To most of us, this is obvious. Yet some people mistakenly grit their teeth and take the attitude that they won't "give in to it," and that trying to use or move the joint will help it recover.

Yet nobody would feel that insisting on using a sore finger will help it. Continued movement of the inflamed tissues will only make them worse.

I am making rather a point of this because in some arthritic conditions, some teeth-gritting may be necessary. I'll explain that presently, but to understand why some painful movement may be necessary in one case and not in another requires you to know what type of ailment is involved.

Bursitis is inclined to develop suddenly. Only by long coincidence would it affect more than one joint at a time. The joint is acutely tender. It becomes red and swollen.

Don't let me give you the idea that these several symptoms provide you with a do-it-yourself method of diagnosis. An acutely painful joint is nothing to tinker with. Diagnosis sometimes is very easy, sometimes it is tricky. Either way, it deserves early treatment if you are to avoid unnecessary suffering.

You will, however, avoid a lot of worry and be better able to co-operate with your doctor if you know something about the main types of joint troubles.

Other joint ailments, or what seem to be joint ailments, may involve sprains, strains, gout, or other troubles. The pain may be in the muscles rather than actually in the joint capsule.

A friend once called me about his wife, who is an artist. She had pains in her arms and shoulders and was terrified because she was sure it was arthritis and that she would have to give up painting.

I told my friend candidly that there was no point in trying to make a diagnosis on the basis of a telephone description, that I strongly doubted that it was arthritis, but if it was or it wasn't, the best thing would be to get his wife to their doctor.

He did. By the next day she was feeling much better and her mind was at ease. She had a not-too-severe bursitis, which responded readily to treatment. The rest of her pains were doubtless nothing but muscular tension, because they disappeared as soon as she relaxed and realized that she wasn't going to be crippled by her imagined "arthritis."

Don't, for several reasons, let the thought of arthritis throw you into a panic. Your nerves can play mean tricks on you, as they did to my friend's wife. For a second reason, differences in ailments call for different treatments. Trying to diagnose your own case can lead you into doing things that may be actually harmful, or at best do you no good. For a third, prompt medical attention means less pain and may mean avoiding the establishment of chronic trouble. Fourth, psychology is vastly important. The patient's frame of mind in real cases of arthritis can be the difference between success and failure in treatment. I have seen it happen.

So find out for sure what your trouble is. Guessing and suffering in silence is the worst thing you can do.

WHAT TO DO ABOUT GOUT

Gout, and its fellow traveler, gouty arthritis, is not going to yield to any of the treatments for the other types of trouble we've discussed.

Gout is a metabolic disorder. The body does not properly use (and get rid of) uric acid, therefore uric acid appears to excess in the blood, and urate crystals can be detected in deposits which gradually form in cartilage and joints.

Attacks of gout come suddenly, and the affected joint becomes hot, red and swollen. It is intensely tender. (Sounds pretty much like the description of bursitis, doesn't it?)

Three-quarters of the time the first attack will be in the big toe, and in most cases, the toe sooner or later is affected. It can attack just about anywhere, however.

The testy and gouty British colonel with his foot propped on a cushion is a worn-out stereotyped character of fiction, but believe me, gout has not disappeared. It is an often-overlooked cause of pain in the joints, particularly when one joint is involved. Once its presence is suspected, laboratory tests readily show the excessive urates. Then you begin to get somewhere with the treatment.

Keep in mind that gout comes suddenly, and that after a period of misery you get over the attack and live in complete comfort, only to have another attack come without warning.

Repeatedly I am asked, "What is the correct diet for gout?" Or, "I have been told to avoid purines. Which foods are high in purines?" Diet is being regarded as of less and less importance in preventing gout—other than that moderation is always a wise rule.

Colchicine, a drug long known for this purpose, is very effective in relieving an attack of gout, but it does nothing at all toward reducing the urate levels, so the basic condition progresses.

However, benemid and other drugs now are proving highly effective in helping the body get rid of uric acid and its derivatives, and I can assure you that diagnosing gout early is important. If too many or too large deposits are allowed to accumulate—which is what happens over a term of years—the trouble becomes chronic.

People who begin getting treatments early, thus preventing the build-up of deposits, go year after year without further attacks.

A good many of them exercise reasonable care with their diet but don't make a fetish of it. The high-purine foods are such things as organ meats (liver, kidney, brains, sweetbreads); the red meats in general; sardines, anchovies, pork, cod and legumes, such as beans, peas.

Lamb, ham, tuna, salmon, crab, oysters and whitefish are of moderate purine content. Eggs, cheese, green vegetables, fruits and most bread and cereals are examples of low-purine foods.

But I repeat: Experience shows that diet is a relatively ineffective way of tackling gout, and the modern drugs for expelling uric acid products are extremely effective. It is a disease primarily of men. Only one patient in twenty or so is a woman.

ARTHRITIS—TWO MAIN TYPES

With actual arthritis it is of utmost significance to distinguish between the two major kinds.

Rheumatoid arthritis isn't just a name for arthritis. It is a particular kind—and a dangerous kind.

It is one of the collagen diseases, or disorders of the connective tissues.

The other big category of arthritis is "degenerative arthritis," also commonly called "osteoarthritis."

While this is, most certainly, an ailment, it is not an acute, identifiable disease as is rheumatoid arthritis. It is a gradual thing, probably best described as part of the natural aging process. Viewing it as simply the result of lifelong wear and tear may be as good an attitude as any.

It is rheumatoid arthritis which cripples people, fusing joints until they are immovable, leaving them with hands that are constricted into claw-shape or immobilizing other parts of the body.

Degenerative arthritis, while painful and progressive in the sense that stiffness gradually increases, need not and, in most cases, does not cripple the individual.

As I said, the psychological attitude of the patient is of great importance—in both types of arthritis.

I shall not soon forget one acute case of rheumatoid arthritis. The patient, a woman, was also stricken with grief and disappointment. In 6 months she changed from a robust, active woman to a miserable cripple.

This should not happen. We must not let it happen. But in a severe case, it is a tremendous battle for both doctor and patient. When the patient loses hope and gives up, prospects are sorry indeed. Listlessness and despair are reflected in the body processes as a whole. This is an important element in almost any illness, and more so with rheumatoid arthritis.

In addition, exercises, physiotherapy and simple movements are painful but necessary. When the patient gives up hope, or becomes generally depressed, there is no will to go on despite the pain, and the battle is lost.

Just what causes rheumatoid arthritis? This we do not know. Many theories have been proposed, but none has yet passed the test of medical and scientific scrutiny.

We can, however, describe the way the disease progresses. First attack is on the synovial membrane, that fluid-containing layer inside the joint capsule.

Along with inflammation of this membrane, and painful swelling, even more dangerous changes are taking place in the bones (which lose their mineral content and become fibrous) and in the cartilage or "bearing" on which the bones ride. The cartilage loses its blood supply and degenerates.

Unless halted, the process ultimately means that the joint becomes completely rigid and immovable. When that time comes, the pain ceases, but the joint is useless.

THE FATE OF THE MUSCLES

Referring back to our earlier discussion of muscle functions: What happens while the joint is being attacked? The pain is such that the muscles become tense and go into spasm. The muscles that flex—those which, in the case of the hand, clench or close the fist—are stronger than the opposing ones, which open the hand.

Hence, the muscle spasm tends to draw the fingers forward. It doesn't draw them into a fist but rather pulls the hand and fingers into a claw-shaped or somewhat hook-like configuration. The opposing muscles, unable to compete, wither from lack of use; in time the stronger ones do so, too.

In the course of the acute phase of the disease, besides the pain and swelling of the joints, the patient has fever, loses weight and may become anemic and chronically tired.

Pain may come and go, or the attack may be pretty much continuous until it has run its course. In fact, no two cases seem to be quite alike. Physician (and patient) must just keep fighting, guiding their efforts by circumstances in the particular case.

Medication (the salicylates are tremendously useful) combats the inflammation. Hormones help temporarily. Gold salts are used with varying success. Sometimes they are very helpful and sometimes not. A certain amount of intelligent trial and error is necessary at times.

It is of great importance to keep the patient's nutrition up to par, and this isn't easy. It may take a lot of coaxing. If the patient recognizes the need and tries to eat even without much appetite, that is a strong step forward. No single food causes or benefits rheumatoid arthritis. There is no special diet for this disorder except a well-balanced, normal one.

The joints, acutely inflamed, must be protected from any additional irritation. This means a great deal of rest, perhaps complete bed rest in some cases. Exercise, in the ordinary sense, is to be limited or avoided. However, to prevent the joints from becoming rigid or "frozen," some movement is required—perhaps only once or twice a day. Here again, every case has to be judged on its own merits. Merely moving an affected joint to its fullest extent in each possible direction tends to prevent the joint from becoming "frozen." However, the joint is permitted to rest most of the time.

Heat, massage and careful nursing play their important parts, too.

Treatment, begun at once, does a great deal to limit or prevent permanent disability. When treatment is delayed, or the patient is unwilling or psychologically unable to fight the disease, the consequences can be severe indeed.

SURGERY HAS ITS USES

In recent years the surgeon, once unable to do anything about rheumatoid arthritis, has come to be important in the correction of some of the resultant deformities. Useless hands now are being straightened, and although the surgery is intricate and difficult, it not only restores appearance but, to varying degrees, brings back their usefulness.

You must expect to find such surgery mainly available in the larger hospitals and medical centers, because it is highly special-ized work, but it is a procedure that a good many people have not yet heard about. Your regular physician can advise you as to where to inquire, or whether it is likely to be of benefit in a par-ticular case.

THE "OTHER KIND OF ARTHRITIS"

Now let's get on with a less grim subject, degenerative arthritis.

The rheumatoid attacks usually come between the ages of 20 and 40, although no age is entirely exempt—not even small chil-dren in some sad cases.

Degenerative arthritis, however, is far more likely to develop in middle age or later—develop to the stage of being noticed, that is. It does not come violently and acutely but creeps along gradu-ally, a "wearing down" matter instead of a savagely destructive one.

The pads of cartilage become thinner, and there is some change in shape of the ends of the bones, with thickening of the edges.

There is good reason to believe that this degenerative process starts about the time we reach our full growth, but that scarcely means that we have arthritis then. Could we compare it, perhaps, to hardening of the arteries? It is part of the long process of grow-ing older.

Some people may begin having rheumatic twinges far earlier than others. Some remain supple and active at 80 or 90. One factor appears to be the quality of the cartilage in the joints. It wears well for some, wears down faster for others.

Injuries we may have entirely forgotten doubtless play their part. So does excess weight, especially in aggravating creakiness of the hips and knees, as well as trouble with the back and feet.

Some of this arthritis is an aftermath of rheumatoid arthritis earlier in life—the joints have been damaged and are going to be somewhat stiffer and uncomfortable.

We certainly must keep in mind, though, that it is entirely up to the individual whether he is going to retain his activity or is going to doom himself to a cane and rocking chair in later life.

A young and attractive secretary once told me she had rheumatoid arthritis in her early twenties. She had been engaged to a fellow who, when he learned of her illness, broke the engagement with the brutal explanation that he "didn't want to be tied down to an invalid."

It might have broken the spirit of some girls, but not this one. It made her mad. She had no visible deformity from the attack, but, as she put it, "My joints were so stiff and painful that it was sheer, utter agony to move in the morning. My doctor told me it was up to me. He'd done all he could do. If I gave in, the joints would get stiffer and stiffer.

"If I just made myself get moving in the morning, I would keep the use of them. Besides, he said, as the day went on, I would find that the pain gradually decreased.

"He was right about it. Sometimes I was tempted to give up, but I just made up my mind that I wouldn't quit. And here I am. It was agony for a while but it has been worth it."

Much the same advice is applicable to people whose arthritis is of wear-and-tear origin rather than caused by active disease. Keep your joints flexible! Don't abuse them by forcing yourself into heavy doses of exercise. This will do no good.

But don't give in to the temptation to stay in bed, or to hobble to a chair and stay there. It will hurt, but keep moving in the morning until you have driven out the stiffness.

Heat will help, and it makes no particular difference whether this is dry heat or any other kind. It's the temperature that helps. A hot soak in the tub, or an electric heating pad—either is good.

What Kind of Medication?

After years of study and restudy, aspirin and its relatives in the drug family, the salicylates, still prove to be the most effective thing to take.

"My doctor," a reader asks, "has had me taking salicylates for several years now. It is usually about six or eight a day. Will this harm me in any way? And should I cut down to prevent the pills from losing their effect from so much use?"

No, it won't harm her to take such reasonable amounts as she needs for comfort, and they usually don't have a diminishing effect. The occasional exception is that some folks find that aspirin irritates the stomach. They may find a buffered form of the drug more satisfactory. Or, for that matter, taking the tablets at meal-time, or even with a glass of milk, often will prevent irritation (the food [or milk] prevents the medicine from irritating the stomach lining).

Cortisone-type medication has had remarkable effect, but it has two qualifications: It is purely temporary (the exact method by which it works is not well known), and on continued use it can lead to a variety of side effects, some of them serious. Taken under your physician's supervision, these medications can be discontinued at any sign of unwanted results. You cannot expect to take them indefinitely.

Resorts featuring special baths are still favored by some arthritis patients, and I certainly have no objection to them. I seriously question some of the explanations as to why some particular kind of water is better for arthritis. The presence of various innocuous salts no doubt helps retain the heat, but I have never been able to find the slightest evidence of any medicinal effect.

However, there are at least two or three other factors involved which I believe to be genuinely helpful:

There is the anticipation of the trip. Get your mind onto something pleasurable and off your aches, and you feel better just from that. Every pain, if you just sit and contemplate it, is worse.

The traveling requires a certain amount of activity, and that works some of the stiffness out.

The psychological lift is an important gain.

Questions about diet for arthritis are hardy perennials. Either I'm being asked what diet I advise, or I'm being quizzed about some trick diet that somebody or other "guarantees."

Aside from a normal, well-balanced diet, there isn't any kind of diet that is going to work miracles. The cartilage pads have become thinner, and the changed shape of the bones makes joints stiffer, and nothing you eat is going to change that—so long as you get adequate nourishment to avoid dietary deficiencies.

Vitamins and mineral supplements won't, either.

Look Out for the Nostrums

Just maintain a healthy suspicion when a "sure cure" is offered. The woods—or should I say the satchels and shelves of the patent-medicine peddlers—are full of all manner of remedies.

A large proportion of them are salicylates, dressed up with fancy labels and fancy prices.

The Arthritis and Rheumatism Foundation has calculated that Americans squander a quarter of a billion dollars a year on quack arthritis treatments and remedies. Some are harmless except that they waste your money. Some are silly. Some probably give quite a lift to the patient so long as he believes or hopes that he is getting over the rheumatism.

Since the discomfort characteristically fluctuates, it is easy for one to be misled, for a time, if he happens to try some new discovery just at the time his joints are feeling easier. Painful joints are common enough and chronic enough, so there is always a supply of new gullible patients to rise to the bait.

You'll save money and get at least as much benefit, and almost always more, by sticking consistently to the few known and inexpensive treatments: heat, salicylates, moderate activity, adequate rest (lie down for a time at midday and in the afternoon, if you can, to take the pressure off your joints) and adequate diet. Keep cheerful, keep interested in other things, and don't confuse all arthritis with the often crippling rheumatoid kind.

As you get on in years, you may become somewhat stiffer, but you aren't going to be incapacitated unless you let it happen.

One final question: "We have heard that the climate in Arizona is perfect, and that arthritis doesn't exist there."

Yes, I've been told of precisely such claims. It's bosh, of course. Arthritis exists there and in any other climate.

All the same, I do know of some people who have found that living in western and southern states can be of substantial benefit. No doubt the warmer weather plays its part. Heat helps! Probably changes in atmospheric pressure have an effect, because some arthritics do get twinges when they feel a storm coming on.

In fairness, however, I must warn you not to get your hopes

too high, not to tear your lives up by the roots and not to risk the expense of finding a new home without keeping in mind that you may be working up to a letdown. An extended visit first will give you a better basis on which to judge any benefits from a climatic or geographic change.

I don't want to discourage anyone from finding a place which may, for him, be more satisfactory, but neither do I want to let anyone in for shattering disappointment when a little caution will prevent it.

The Back and the Extremities

Arthritis, as well as other joint troubles, can affect *any* joint, and that includes those formed by the 24 bones in the spine: the pelvic bones and others.

A certain amount of spinal arthritis is by no means uncommon, and a good many people encounter some between the cervical vertebrae (the bones of the neck).

Since nerves to different parts of the body branch out from the spinal cord and must pass between the vertebrae, the arthritic changes in the bones can exert pressure on some of these nerves.

This is the simple explanation of some of the "mysterious" numbness, tingling or even pain in fingers, arms and shoulders. X rays of the neck sometimes reveal arthritic changes, and the patient wonders why the doctor wants those X rays for troubles that seem to be in the arms or hands.

"I wake up every morning with my hands asleep. The tingling is a terrible nuisance until I have been up a while," one woman said. "Then I'm all right for the rest of the day, but the following morning I go through it all again."

With variations, this has been the story from a great many people. If the situation isn't severe, but mostly an annoyance, I often suggest the least expensive remedy I know: Try changing your sleeping position. Try a larger pillow, or two pillows. Or try sleeping with no pillow at all. You'd be surprised how many times this puts an end to the complaint.

Where such referred pain is severe and intractable, stronger measures may be needed—a neck or spinal brace perhaps. In other cases, a device for applying neck traction once or twice a day (perhaps morning and evening) will help to separate the bones enough to take the pressure off the nerve.

In very severe cases, adjacent vertebrae may sometimes be fused (fastened rigidly together with bone grafts). Movement, of course, is lost at that particular point, but the nerves are permanently relieved of pressure or irritation there.

THE MISNAMED "SLIPPED" DISC

I'm not sure where the term *slipped disc* came from, but either *ruptured* or *damaged* would be a better term. Rarely does the disc (cushion of cartilage between two vertebrae) really slip. Rather, it may be crushed or made lopsided or otherwise be damaged. It is generally the result of an injury, a sitting fall often being involved.

A conservative approach to this type of injury is usually preferable. Girdles, braces, traction and, sometimes, appropriate exercises often bring satisfactory results. Again, when none of these will serve, surgery is the court of last appeal. Sometimes it is necessary, but I recommend a wait-and-see attitude while the conservative treatments are tried first.

Do not leap to the conclusion that backache means disc trouble. At least 80 percent of backaches are due to muscular spasm or strain brought on by a sudden twist, or fall or the strain of lifting. Muscles may be stretched or torn; the attaching tendons may be strained. Once such an injury has occurred, a repetition is more likely to occur, and from less stress.

The very complex pattern of muscles in the back can make it difficult to tell at first just what position subjects you to strain on the damaged place. It will be worth your while to keep watch of the positions in which a twinge occurs. Once you have that position or movement (reaching, lifting, turning, whatever it is) pegged in your mind, you can make a conscious effort to avoid strain in that position. It will pay off in avoiding further damage.

For another precaution, recall to mind some of your early

lessons about posture. If any single thing must absorb major blame for backaches, it is poor posture. The central column of the body, the spine, is a flexible column of 24 "blocks" or vertebrae. Kept properly piled one atop another, they carry the weight easily.

But let them tip out of alignment, and severe stress is placed on the muscles that have to keep trying to hold the spine back in position. So if you have back troubles, start conscientiously trying to sit and stand straight. Stop slouching. Stand on your two feet; don't let yourself stand hipshot.

For a special kind of backache—waking up in the morning with an ache that gradually diminishes after you've been up and around —suspect your bed. You may be sleeping on too soft a mattress and spring.

Yes, too soft. Rarely is a bed too hard. Some people find the trouble vanishing when they get a new spring or a firmer mattress. But others have equal success at trivial cost by slipping a bed board between springs and mattress. A sheet of plywood a few feet square makes a very simple bed board.

PAIN IN THE LOWER BACK

Low back pain, a frequent complaint to me and to most physicians (except those in totally unrelated specialties), is one of the more ornery problems, medically speaking.

Sometimes it is most difficult to persuade a patient that he (or she) ought to forget about pills, braces or therapy, and instead lose 25 or 30 pounds, start standing up straight and begin getting a reasonable amount of exercise every day.

Add to this the fact that nervous tension, and consequently hypertense back muscles, can be part of the picture. Just try to convince some patients of this! They prefer, for what reason I'm not sure, to insist that they must have kidney trouble or a slipped disc, or—well, you name it.

It's a waste of time and money, in the majority of chronic cases of low back pain, to start X-raying and so on until the patient has given the obvious methods a fair trial. But if we've spent 20 or 30 or 40 or more years developing sloppy posture and a paunch, it isn't as easy as it sounds to change our habits. Calling it "lumbago" doesn't get us anywhere. Knowing how often the common faults are responsible will get a lot of us somewhere.

Prostate disease in men can cause referred back pain; in women, pelvic disorders are very frequently blamed—but they are far less often involved than is thought.

One special kind of back pain, sciatica, may not be helped by simple methods. The sciatic muscle is a large one which sends a branch down the back of each thigh.

The pain is in the legs, or in part of the back or hips, and the legs. The usual cause is one which we have already discussed in other matters—pressure on the nerve.

It is true that some infection or other form of nerve involvement may be causing the sciatic nerve to send out its pain signals. But the pinching often is at the spine, and girdling, traction, and the other things we have already discussed are the effective answer, in many cases, to sciatica.

In the complicated human body there are, naturally, all sorts of variants of the ailments we've been discussing, and there are some that we haven't touched upon at all—but an entire book, let alone a single chapter, wouldn't be large enough to cover every possibility.

It is my hope, however, that this chapter has given you a sound and useful understanding of why and how some of our skeletal and muscular troubles come about and thus has provided you with a good deal of know-how in contending with them or, best of all, avoiding them.

11

HORMONES, HEALTH AND HOKUM

MAXIM 11 *Respect the uses—and dangers—of hormones, some of them necessary for life itself.*

Let's start with the word *gland.*

What is a gland? It's an organ, usually relatively small and sometimes very small, that secretes or excretes some material or other.

Secrete has more than one meaning. It can mean to hide or conceal. In the sense we use it, it means to put together or create something for inner use. So a gland secretes useful material.

Other glands excrete, meaning that they get rid of some deleterious substance.

We are equipped with countless little glands, such as the sebaceous, oil-giving glands of the skin, the sweat glands and a variety of glands in the mucous membranes. If our noses run, it is the work of glands providing fluid to counteract irritation. If we are in danger, our adrenal glands fire forth adrenalin, which speeds up our hearts and in many ways helps us muster our vigor and alertness to meet the emergency. If we have an infection, the lymph glands filter out wastes and poisons that the blood has carried from the site of infection.

Many glands operate at what we might call the local level—the skin glands, those that provide mucus, and so on.

Others secrete materials that exercise regulatory control over parts of the body distant from the gland. These secretions we call "hormones."

We are all familiar, I am sure, with the term *endocrine glands,* although we may not have stopped to ask what the term means.

The endocrine glands produce secretions for internal use, that is to say, the secretions pass directly into the blood stream.

Our "exocrine glands," on the other hand, release their materials to a surface, either the surface of the skin or another surface, as saliva is released to the inner surfaces of the mouth, and enzymes and digestive juices to the surfaces of the stomach or intestine.

The pancreas, which will be discussed further in another chapter, combines the two types of activity. It discharges into the digestive canal a fluid that aids in digesting carbohydrates, protein and fat—its exocrine activity. Another part of the pancreas sends insulin into the blood stream—endocrine.

The insulin originates in small units called the "islets of Langerhans." However, there are two types of these islets, called *alpha* and *beta.* The alpha cells produce glucagon, a hormone which serves to raise the blood-sugar level. The beta islets produce insulin, which lowers it.

I wouldn't bother with these technicalities except to try to illustrate how very complicated the glands and their products become, and to ask you to keep in mind the word *regulate.*

These hormones from the pancreas work in two directions: one type raising, the other lowering the amount of blood sugar. This *maintaining of a balance* seems to be one of the most basic rules of Nature. Balance is the thing. Too little of something may starve us; too much of the same thing poison us.

This axiom quite frequently has to be pointed out by physicians to people who become too intent about medicines. "If one pill is good for me, two ought to be twice as good," these people argue—and sometimes come to grief. And the same with vitamins: People who are getting (or should be getting, if they would eat the right things) enough vitamins, insist on taking extra vitamins. This is wasteful. Happily, within reason it does no harm, although it is possible to cause vitamin poisoning by excessive amounts of some. Others are simply discharged by the body when too much is taken in.

Hormones, extremely powerful materials, cannot be employed with such casual impunity.

PITUITARY—THE "BOSS GLAND"

The endocrine hormones are fascinating. They control such matters as our growth, appearance, activity, reproduction and personality.

Many of them are interrelated; others operate with comparative independence.

The pituitary gland, the master gland of the system, is so important that Nature has encased it within the strong protection of the skull. It alone secretes at least half a dozen hormones serving various purposes, either directly or indirectly. It governs, for example, the activity of the important thyroid, genital and adrenal glands.

Decrease the effective activity of the pituitary, and the consequences can be such as infertility, lassitude, small stature, low blood sugar and dwarfism. Increase it excessively and acromegaly or gigantism can result.

Removal or destruction of the pituitary means that some means must be found to replace the various hormones normally produced by all the endocrine glands controlled by the pituitary.

Since I mentioned growth (gigantism or dwarfism as the extremes), perhaps we'd best point out that this does not mean that we can tinker with the pituitary and govern how big we are to be. There are, we know, other factors involved. At the proper time in life, as we come to the end of our increase in height, a change takes place in the ends of the long bones of the body. Excessive amounts of the growth hormone from the pituitary (somatotrophin) can speed up growth or cause abnormal growth prior to that time. Too little can result in dwarfism.

But too much of the hormone after that time leads to acromegaly—the long bones do not continue to grow, but the face, feet, hands and soft tissues of the body continue to grow. This, obviously, leads to monstrosity.

Researchers are also cautious because some factor which has a diabetes-producing consequence is attached to this hormone, or perhaps part of it.

Hormones are powerful substances, chemically intricate and physiologically difficult because of the interaction between them; they are not to be trifled with.

They have been the tool of overoptimistic dreamers, and I have no doubt that this will continue. Some of the claims made for hormones have been sheer hokum. Some no doubt have been sincere but have been based on too little understanding of their nature.

Replenishing hormones of some kinds to compensate for deficiencies is practicable and successful. Retarding overactivity of some glands is a necessity.

But the purpose is to restore, as accurately as we can, the *normal* level. Do not be misled by wishful thinking or by glowing claims that hormones can produce this or that seeming miracle.

Health isn't a matter of miracles. Health derives from maintaining our bodies in a state that Nature, at her best, intends.

THE THYROID, AN AMENABLE GLAND

Perhaps to many readers, the word *hormones* has taken on the overtone of meaning sex hormones. Various sex hormones exist, and they are highly useful, but they are only part of the picture.

Let's start with the well-known thyroid, which is one of the endocrine glands, important to us day by day and hour by hour. It also is proving to be amenable to correction when it gets a bit off stride.

It lies close to the "Adam's apple" but exerts its influence all over the body.

Somebody once coined the name "chemical messengers" for hormones. They carry the signals. They guide. They regulate. If you recall your high school chemistry, they act as catalysts. They don't participate in a chemical reaction by becoming a physical part of it, but the reactions of other chemicals do not occur without their presence.

Very small amounts are required. The gland itself weighs less than one ounce. The thyroid happens to be the only gland that produces hormones containing iodine. The amount of iodine is very small, however. One scientist, groping for a way to describe how small this trace is, said it would be about the amount of iodine a person would absorb by sniffing the cork of a bottle of iodine once a day.

This also offers a gauge of how little of the hormone is needed to do its chores.

Let the amount of thyroid activity fall below normal and a person slows down physically and mentally, is tired, is unusually sensitive to cold and develops dry and puffy skin.

Overactive thyroid goads the individual into a great deal of activity and beyond, into nervousness, tremors, sweating, restlessness and sometimes palpitation and such symptoms.

The physician's (and sometimes the surgeon's) goal is to do all that is possible to restore the thyroid to normal activity. Not too much. Not too little.

Yet even here I find people who ask for thyroid for some secondary purpose. One female reader asked:

Dear Doctor:

I have tried all kinds of diets but I just can't seem to reduce. A friend of mine has been getting thyroid pills from her doctor and has lost about 20 pounds. How much do you think would be right for me to take?

It is true enough that some low-thyroid individuals put on weight from the combination of lack of activity and too much eating. Some! Not all. It is equally possible for one to be inactive because of thyroid deficiency, yet to eat suitably and not put on weight.

In other words, these are two separate problems. One is thyroid regulation. The other is diet regulation. One may at times help correct the other, but it certainly does *not* mean that artificial stimulation of the thyroid is a safe or effective way to reduce. I hope the woman understood my explanation when I told her I could certainly not sanction any such performance.

When the thyroid is genuinely underactive, giving thyroid material by mouth corrects the situation.

Reducing overactivity is not always that easy. Some drugs that can help are known, but in other cases surgical removal of part of the gland has been necessary.

Where increased activity brings reduction of weight, that is an incidental, although very useful, by-product. Besides restored energy, there may be other benefits, such as brighter eyes, correction of sparse hair growth and sometimes remarkable brightening of the whole personality.

How to Spot Thyroid Trouble

The symptoms I've mentioned for too much or too little thyroid activity are the principal ones that the patient will be able to see.

There are very exact ways of testing, once this trouble is suspected.

The thyroid, dubbed "the gyroscope of metabolism," is tested more or less approximately by measuring the metabolic rate—the rate at which we use up the food we eat. This, in turn, is reflected by the rate at which we use oxygen, since one depends upon the other.

Hence the BMR, or basal metabolism rate, is significant. Its determination is a morning procedure of having the patient eat nothing, lie quietly for a time and then breathe through a tube so that we can measure the amount of oxygen used in a specified time.

Even more precision is afforded by the PBI, or protein-bound iodine test, a blood analysis. Since the thyroid hormones are the only ones containing iodine, and the iodine atoms are tied to protein molecules, measuring the amount of such "bound" iodine measures the quantity of hormone.

Thyroid imbalance can occur at any age. Among the elderly I have found thyroid deficiency to be a not uncommon problem, not severe, perhaps, but a subtle cause of "feeling cold" to a greater degree than age alone would cause.

It can occur in early infancy or even sooner (before a child is born) and have terrible consequences—cretinism (a very severe form of mental retardation accompanied by physical changes).

When, as is increasingly frequent now, this condition is recognized immediately, babies can be treated so successfully that they grow up as perfectly normal children instead of deformed mental cripples. The basic reason, of course, may be a faulty pituitary that does not incite the thyroid to adequate activity.

Before we leave the topic, let's at least mention goiter.

It is a declining ailment, but it has not disappeared, and there is no reason to expect that it will, entirely.

Since the thyroid needs iodine, trouble commences if for a long period there is not enough iodine to supply even the small traces required. There is little or no iodine in the soil in some areas—the Great Lakes region, the Pacific Northwest, and various other regions of the world. There we had the "goiter belts." Where people got a good deal of sea food, there was little goiter because the sea is rich in iodine.

With lack of iodine, the thyroid gland tries to make up for it by working harder—by enlarging. It may or may not succeed in compensating. If lack of iodine is too great, no amount of effort by the body can produce enough of the hormone. And less than one-thousandth of an ounce is the average amount in the body!

In the last several decades use of iodized salt has become so general that goiter from this cause is vanishing.

Goiter can develop from other causes, however. Tumors of the thyroid may develop, more often in later life. There may be one or several such nodules. About 3 percent either are or become malignant, and the likelihood favors this among the single- rather than multiple-nodule cases. A tumor in a young person warrants special suspicion on this score.

For health, then, examine and, in some cases, keep continuing watch over a thyroid growth.

PARATHYROIDS AND OTHER GLANDS

The parathyroid glands, usually four in number, are little bean-shaped organs near the thyroid. The parathyroids, unlike most of the endocrine glands, are not governed by the autocratic pituitary. Likewise, the parathyroids are not very likely to come much into the field of interest for the average person, but they are important.

The parathyroids govern the body's utilization of calcium, the rate at which it is withdrawn from the bones and then replaced, and probably the withdrawal of it from connective tissues, also.

Too rapid withdrawal causes brittleness and fractures, but keeping the diet very high in calcium can minimize this.

If the gland is underactive, cramps, muscular disorders, and possibly convulsions can result; there is a distinct tendency toward cataracts. Extract of the parathyroid hormone is of help only temporarily, but very large doses of Vitamin D, and sometimes the use of other medication, is a dependable treatment.

The thymus is a curious gland, apparently intended by Nature to protect children from disease, but the exact process, not well understood, is posing some neat questions for the research people who are gradually exacting some parts of the answer. Unlike other glands, the thymus ceases activity in the early teens and atrophies.

For whatever reason, it seems to have an effect on patients with myasthenia gravis, a disease involving extreme muscle weakness. Removal of the thymus has helped some of them. Since removal seems to have no ill effect on health, it is considered worth doing in such cases.

There are still other glands. Although some, like the thymus, do not abide by all of the presumed "rules" for endocrine glands they nonetheless are part of the whole delicate regulatory pattern. There is, for example, the hypothalamus, a part of the brain but so responsive to elements in the endocrine system as to give us reason to include it as a "gland" if we choose. Its functions are in the control of body temperature, sleep and appetite—all, for the most part, in the realm outside conscious control.

It is not likely that very many readers ever will have trouble with the last three glands that we've been discussing, but it seems worthwhile to include them as further examples of the immense regulatory services of the endocrine system and its ramifications.

In fact, the endocrine glands generally are amazingly dependable, particularly when you remember what an enormous number of functions they govern, the tremendously small physical volume of the hormones, and the intricacy of their interactions.

The Wonderful Adrenals

If you are exposed to sudden danger, or are seriously wounded, a couple of important little glands, one perched atop each kidney, come to your instant aid.

They are the adrenals.

You know the medical value of adrenalin. It is another name for epinephrin, which is but one of the materials secreted by the adrenals.

In time of anger or danger, the output of these glands speeds up our breathing and heart rate, boosts blood pressure, releases stored sugar into the blood (for energy) and gives us the extra vigor and self-confidence to do what we have to do.

Yet adrenalin is only one of more than two dozen hormones that have been identified as originating in these glands.

Another entire family of hormones comes from the upper part of the glands, or the adrenal cortex. These are the cortisone-type (or corticoid) hormones, which have the widest imaginable regulatory interests.

They lay the groundwork for sex hormone production, control excretion of minerals and salt and potassium, control sugar output and, indeed, have other tasks that we know are involved even though we do not understand just how. The effect of cortisone in ailments of the joints, some skin conditions and a variety of other matters is very widely known.

Occasionally someone notes that ACTH is sometimes used, and on other occasions cortisone (or hydrocortisone or other variants). "Are they the same thing?" they ask.

No, not at all—although the end result may be. For ACTH (*a*drenocortico*t*rophic *h*ormone) is produced naturally by the pituitary, our far-reaching "boss gland." It is the "chemical messenger" that tells the adrenals to release more cortisone. Hence, whether the doctor gives ACTH or cortisone, a similar end result comes of it. (Yes, there are fine points which are considered in deciding whether to use one or the other.)

Failure of the adrenals to function adequately is called Addison's disease. It involves weakness, low blood pressure, low blood sugar, loss of sexual potency, shock and change in color (bronzing) of the skin.

Overactivity (as from tumors of the adrenals or from hyperactivity of the pituitary) is called Cushing's syndrome, which may have such symptoms as increased blood pressure, excessive hair growth or virilization (exaggerated male characteristics, or masculinization in women) and sugar in the urine.

Neither is a frequent disease; both can be treated these days, although it wasn't so very many years ago that we hadn't yet traced enough of the obscure causes to know what to do.

Sex Hormones—Two Kinds

The sex hormones, as you have gathered already, overlap the work of other hormones. Low thyroid activity can contribute to lack of fertility, although the thyroid isn't a sex gland. Secretions of the pituitary and adrenals play parts in sexual functions or the so-called "secondary sex characteristics."

Why does the male grow taller and heavier and more ruggedly muscled than the female? This goes back to the control exercised by the pituitary.

The endocrine system is so interrelated that it does not come apart in neat, compartmented sections. A lack of understanding this interrelationship permitted the great excitement, quite some years ago, over some fine-sounding nonsense about using "monkey glands" to restore youthful vigor to people who weren't young any more.

Today you see various products boasting that they contain hormones and ostensibly can perform all sorts of wonders. But it just isn't that simple.

But let's get on with the sex hormones, which are of the androgenic (male) type and the estrogenic (female) type.

This does not mean that all of them are limited to a person of one sex or the other. The sex glands produce some of each type. The female hormone leads numerically in the female, and male hormone predominates in the male, but there probably is no such thing as being "completely" male or female.

But some aspects, naturally, are entirely different. The male hormone, testosterone, from the testes, has to do with various processes, among them the development of the male sperm and seminal fluid.

Deficiency of the hormone not only means low or absent productivity of sperm but will result in development of feminine features or characteristics.

It also plays its part in a condition known as cryptorchism or "undescended testicle."

At birth, the testicles are up inside the abdomen; later they ordinarily descend into the scrotum. When they do not, there are several consequences. Ultimately they will atrophy; in any case, they cannot function because the temperature inside the body is too high—the purpose of the scrotum is to get them outside of the body, where the temperature is low enough to suit the tissues which produce sperm. Finally, there is a slight risk that the undescended testicles may in time become cancerous.

Men: Have you ever noticed that in cold weather the scrotum is snug to the body, and in hot weather or after a hot bath the bag is hanging much lower? This is Nature's mechanism to keep the testes at proper temperature. This can be observed in boy babies.

A Case of Needless Worry

I have had a great number of letters about undescended testicle because people don't hear much about it unless it happens in their immediate family.

The matter can be corrected. It is well to wait until the boy is about 10 years old; often it is only a question of delay, and normal development comes about without any treatment.

Between 10 and 14, however, it is time to give Nature some help. Injection of hormones takes care of the whole problem in many cases.

In at least one case the parents were much alarmed at this, and wrote to me:

We have heard of cases of hormones causing boys to take
on girlish characteristics, and we are very doubtful whether
we should take this chance with our son, who is a thorough
boy in every way except for this trouble with the testicles.

In the first place, the condition obviously has to be corrected,
because the boy will be sterile if both testes are undescended. If
one is down, fertility may not be impaired.

In the second place, the hormones used for this purpose will
not and cannot cause feminization. The hormone secreted by the
anterior part of the pituitary is injected—another example of the
pituitary stimulating glands in distant parts of the body. In this
case, it encourages more action by the male sex glands, and there
is no possibility of what the parents feared.

So you see why, if endocrine problems are to make any sense,
it is necessary to realize the multiplicity of glands and hormones.
Just saying "hormones" doesn't mean much unless you know what
kind of hormones are involved.

(Just to finish the story of undescended testicle, if the hormone
treatment does not succeed, one can always resort to surgery—a
sure means of correcting the condition. It makes sense, though,
and saves expense to try the other ways first.)

HORMONES AND MALIGNANCIES

There is also a widespread misapprehension about the relationship between hormones and cancer. It is quite true that in
some instances hormones have a decided effect on the growth of
cancer. This is not the same thing as saying that hormones cause
cancer.

Take, for example, breast cancer. If this occurs in pregnancy,
when the endocrine system is extremely active, the cancer grows
with great rapidity, and the closest medical attention is necessary.
The same cancer, occurring at any other time, would progress
more slowly.

It is thus obvious, I think, that the hormonal activity doesn't
cause the cancer, else breast cancer would be frequent in time of
pregnancy. As a matter of fact, it is not.

For another example, cancer of the prostate (and the prostate is itself a gland) often can be slowed down tremendously by giving estrogenic hormones—in a sense, "neutralizing" the natural male hormones by introducing female hormones.

Continued use of such hormones in a man, even in one well along in life, can cause chest tissues to grow abnormally and foster development of other somewhat feminine characteristics. Stopping or reducing the hormones reverses the process.

These are other applications of the same sort of treatment. The combination of hormones and X ray has been used successfully in advanced cases of breast cancer. I do not mean that these cases have been cured. Surgical removal, as soon as possible, is the only known method of combatting breast cancer. In cases that have already progressed beyond the stage for surgery, the disease can be slowed down by the removal of ovaries to eliminate the influence of estrogen. Some women who were virtual invalids have put on weight, have regained energy and have been able to do their housework for quite some time because of such treatments, even though, in the end, the disease was beyond stopping. Still, it afforded added life, comfort and usefulness.

Thus the growing understanding of hormones is achieving results that would have been utterly unbelievable only a few decades ago. It may be that a few more decades will add new uses which will be just as wonderful.

However, daydreaming isn't of any benefit to us now. Understanding the nature of hormones, and knowing something about what is possible with their use (along with an awareness of the sort of claims that are not factual), give us more means of promoting our total health.

HORMONES AND THE FEMALE SYSTEM

The female hormones are the counterpart in women of the male hormones in men—plus.

The ovaries secrete hormones that control, for many years, the release each month of an ovum or egg. Other hormones regulate such things as lactation (production of milk), the menstrual cycle

and a considerable number of subsidiary aspects of motherhood—
the muscular activity of the uterus, which must prepare for the
process of childbearing, is one example of this.

Estradiol is the principal hormone of the estrogen group; others
are modifications of it or actuated by it. A second important
female hormone is progesterone, which comes to prominence once
pregnancy has commenced.

Without going into boring detail, the reliable method of de-
termining pregnancy in its early stages is dependent upon the
alteration of hormones. The speed with which this alteration occurs after pregnancy has begun illustrates the sensitivity and
basic importance of the endocrine system. As a consequence,
pregnancy tests may be positive very soon after fertilization of
the egg.

In time (around the age of 45, or a few years less or half a
dozen years more) the ovaries cease functioning. No more ova,
or eggs, appear as the recipient of fertilization and the start of
pregnancy. The hormonal secretions of the ovaries dwindle and
cease. This is menopause or "the change of life."

How does the endocrine system keep track of time with such
relative accuracy over something like 30 years? How does it
regulate the repeated process of menstruation? Why does it shape
women thus and men so? Why do men grow beards and get bald?
Why do women cry easily or become ecstatic with a baby in their
arms?

I don't know the answers to all these things. If it takes a hundred miles of understanding, the researchers are moving ahead a
foot here and an inch there. They've come a long way. When I
have time I sometimes sit back and marvel at how *much* they
have discovered about questions that once seemed beyond solving, and I lose a little patience with people who complain because, therefore, we don't yet know it all.

Or am I being querulous?

Quite a number of hitherto insoluble difficulties now can be
eased or corrected by what has been laboriously learned about
the glands and hormones.

Many millions of people are being helped. I am thinking of one
very large group, women in menopause who suffer (and suffer at

times is a pretty mild word for it) the hot flashes, tensions and nerves that accompany the drastic change when hormones of a certain kind cease being secreted, and the system has to adapt itself to operating with a different pattern of hormones.

Over hundreds and thousands of years, women have had to struggle through this upsetting period. Some did it easily. Some agonized through it. It is only in the last few years that we have been able to give them hormones for, say, 6 months or a year, to make the transition easier.

This is wonderful.

But what bothers me is the notion, fostered and used by commercial interests, that hormones therefore can be indiscriminately peddled for all sorts of things.

I am bombarded, until I want to plug my ears, by women who want to know whether "hormone creams" can increase their bust measurement by two inches. By balding people who think that some "hormone salve" will give them bushy hair. By women who want to know whether face cream with "hormones" will eliminate wrinkles and give them complexions that belong to girls of 17.

None of these appealing concepts has any practical or scientific reason for acceptance, so far as I have been able to discover—and believe me, I've tried to find out about them.

The word *hormone* has acquired a magic. Using hormones within the limits of our knowledge can do great things for us, but trying to use this mighty influence for such purposes as providing bigger bustlines, more hair or schoolgirl skin smacks a little too much of using a shotgun to kill a mouse or resorting to prayer for rain so that we won't have to sprinkle the lawn tomorrow.

Your doctor has both training and a powerful recognition of the power of hormones. It is his profession to know these things. Let him decide when to use them. If he can't, who can?

But maintain a suspicious caution about "hormone products" that you can buy—and are eloquently urged to buy—without prescription. For the most part, they will have such slight hormone content as to have no detectable effect, except to get you to spend money. Sometimes, however, they can harm you. Hormones of some types can be absorbed through the skin. I have in mind one case of which I had personal knowledge: a man who used a hormone preparation for baldness and presently became impotent and began to exhibit feminine characteristics. Depending upon the type of hormone and the sex of the user, such things can happen.

Hormones can be immensely valuable but are safe only when handled by those who know how to use them, what to expect, and what to watch for in the way of unwanted consequences.

12

REVITALIZE
YOUR VITAL ORGANS

MAXIM 12 *Give your internal organs a chance—or at least half a chance—to do a good job for you, and they will.*

There are two or three interesting and useful lessons to pick out of the following letter.

It rather shocked me, in a way, to receive it, because it was written by an obviously fluent and intelligent person. And yet—well, here's the letter.

Dear Sir:

If you would care to write about the following, I would appreciate it.

1. Describe a gall bladder attack.
2. What brings on such an attack?
3. How can one avoid an attack?

Two co-workers, self-styled medical authorities after reading a couple of magazine articles, insist that this what I have once or twice a year.

I would like to explain my background. I have been vomiting for years, and my family doctor always said it was a case of nerves. My father was very mild-mannered and my mother is a high-strung, emotional person, as well as a perfectionist.

My younger brother is a very mild-mannered person who
to my knowledge has never had a case of nerves. The rest of
us in the family have had this vomiting for years. Whether
we are considered high-strung by our friends and relatives,
I do not know.

Since I have just had another vomiting spell, I would like
to know more about gall bladder attacks.

What shocks me is that the writer of the letter, while clearly
aware that her advisers are "self-styled medical authorities," puts
enough stock in their home-made theories to want to "know more
about gall bladder attacks."

Certainly I don't object to having people learn more about the
way their bodies operate! I'm in favor of it. I spend a great deal
of my time on that very thing—explaining to people.

But when somebody accumulates a very little knowledge (and
of a shaky sort to boot) and then tries to jam down some friend's
throat the idea that a "diagnosis" has been made, it's time to
protest.

When nearly an entire family has been vomiting periodically
for years, and the family's doctor already has pegged it as a nervous reaction, doesn't it become pretty silly to begin arguing that
it must, instead, be "gall bladder attacks" in one of these nervous
people?

I repeat: The more sound information about health that we
can transmit to the public, the better. But it's up to the individual
to use that information within the bounds of common sense. Seems
to me this is particularly true if he starts trying out his notions
on somebody else.

Trying to diagnose a gall bladder attack on the basis of an
article or two, when it takes very close to 10 years of education
after high school to produce a qualified young doctor, just doesn't
make sense.

In any event, a physician doesn't snatch some snap-judgment
guess as to what *might* ail a patient and then try to prove that
that's it.

Instead, he first gathers all the information he can from the
patient. What exactly is troubling him? What is his background?

How long has the trouble persisted, and under what circumstances?

Then he adds to this such general data as are available from a physical examination. What factors are normal? Are some abnormal?

Then it is time enough to narrow things down to specific tests for ailments that fit the facts.

A comparatively small number of symptoms appear over and over again—but in different patterns. The single symptom, like vomiting in this case, rarely means very much by itself. Vomiting may be from nervous tension, excitement, gastritis, poisoning, intestinal obstruction and a good many other causes.

The smart thing is to know what symptoms deserve being diagnosed by a physician—and then letting him do it.

We'll return, presently, to the gall bladder, but let's first take a longer view of the internal organs generally, and the matter of caring for them—the specialty called "internal medicine."

Interns and Internists

Some people still are confused over the difference between an intern and an internist, and perhaps it's too bad such similar terms are used for such different meanings.

When a medical student graduates from medical school he is not yet ready to start practice on his own. He must still have a year of work under supervision. This is his year spent in a hospital as an intern. He is encouraged to decide what needs to be done and how to go at it, but his decisions on important matters must be confirmed by the senior physicians. It is a year of transition, of transfer from learning things into the task of learning how to apply the knowledge.

At the end of that year he is ready for full licensing.

He may go into practice then.

Or he may, instead, remain at that same or some other hospital for two, three or more years as a "resident." He is a full-fledged physician, learning to specialize in some field, under the direction and teaching of certified specialists.

It may be pediatrics, orthopedics, obstetrics, surgery or nearly a score of others.

One of these specialties is internal medicine, and when the training is complete and the resident has passed rigorous examinations required by the specialty boards, he becomes a certified internist (specialist in internal medicine).

Trying to define exactly what he does is somewhat baffling. He isn't a surgeon, psychiatrist or eye specialist. He doesn't deal with a limited area or field, as does the dermatologist (skin), ear-nose-throat specialist or urologist.

The internist, like the pediatrician, deals with any part of the body that requires treatment. But he does not engage in surgery. He is an expert diagnostician, and he may, in some cases, concentrate on a subspecialty, directing his attention primarily to the heart or some other organ.

We've discussed the heart, respiratory and digestive systems by themselves, so now let's consider some of the other internal organs that are especially important cogs in our human machine, the body.

For practical and medical purposes we consider the internal organs to be those of the abdomen, with the exception of the genital organs which involve separate specialties. Thus we'll be discussing the liver, gall bladder, pancreas and the like.

WHY THE APPEAL FOR "LIVER PILLS"?

It has often puzzled me as to how the appeal of "liver pills" or "kidney pills" ever managed to gain such a widespread hold on the public imagination. It's somewhat easier to understand the lure of "digestion pills," although we've already been over that— the fact that there isn't any particular medication that is automatically helpful in this regard, any more than there's any patent "tonic" that is "good for you no matter what ails you."

The truth is, I guess, that some people just like to take some sort of medicine with the fond belief that they are doing themselves some good, even if they don't know what purpose the potion is supposed to be serving, and quite often don't even know what, if anything, is the matter.

Why, with equal logic, shouldn't people take "Pat's Patent Pancreas Pills" or some equally ridiculous catchpenny trap? Perhaps because they just haven't heard very much about the pancreas, even though the number of people with an ailment of the pancreas (think of the millions with diabetes!) probably exceeds by far the number who ever have real trouble with the liver or some of the other organs.

The best rule I can think of for not wasting money on patent medicines is never to take any unless you know exactly what you are taking it for, and what it is supposed to do for you.

In practice, this may come pretty close to saying that you'll be better off never to take any medicine unless your doctor prescribes it, but I am trying to leave enough of a loophole to admit the use of some things that, technically, are patent medicines but have their useful place. For aspirin, used within reason and in its various modifications, is helpful to most of us for incidental headaches and in easing the discomfort of flu or colds, or casual muscular pains.

Foot powders, and salves for minor irritations, sunburn lotions, baby powders, mild laxatives (when used with discretion), household antiseptics—all these and a good many more are "patent medicines," but they have their uses.

What I warn against is the habit of deciding that you have some illness or other and then buying patent medicines just because the label happens to mention that ailment. Or mentions the organ that you suspect is involved.

These remedies, for the most part, are relatively harmless, because the Food and Drug Administration insists on prescriptions for the more potent drugs. In some instances a very small quantity of a drug may be permitted in a patent remedy. This, however, means that if a "remedy" is safe enough to be sold without prescription, it is likewise so medically feeble as to have scant value, especially if you have an ailment of genuine danger.

No doubt, in some instances, taking excessive amounts of these remedies can do some damage, but the most important reason for avoiding them is that you can lull yourself, for a time anyway, into a false sense of security. To put it another way, too many times a person finally goes to a doctor only when a condition has progressed so far as to be difficult to treat.

If people who habitually buy patent medicines would instead spend half as much, or even one-tenth as much on an occasional visit to their doctors, they could avoid some serious illnesses and besides that be able to spend the difference on furniture or some new clothes.

The "Great Protector," the Liver

The blood sometimes is called "the great protector" because of the multiple tasks it performs.

The liver is an equally great protector.

It plays a part in blood formation, involving the clotting ability of the blood, for one thing. It stores iron and traces of copper that are necessary in formation of red cells in the blood. It also stores Vitamin A. Starch (in the form of glycogen) is stored in the liver, ready to be released in the form of sugar when we need it. It has a detoxifying function—that is, it removes poisons. It likewise removes ammonia and other by-products of protein metabolism.

And it makes bile and releases it to the digestive tract, where it is an important factor in digestion of fats in particular.

With such a complex group of tasks, is it any wonder that I warn people against supposing that some sort of patent medicine could automatically be good for the liver?

The liver is best left alone unless some specific illness develops; then it needs most skilful diagnosis and treatment. The liver, given a chance, has remarkable recuperative powers, however.

The primary threat against the proper functioning of the liver is infection. Hepatitis leaps to mind first (contaminated water and food supplies are one cause). Another form of hepatitis is homologous serum jaundice, which can be passed from one person to another by a blood transfusion. This is one reason for our strict concern over the health of blood donors. A person who has had hepatitis should not donate blood.

Cirrhosis—a virtual hardening due to scarring of cells of the liver—long has been associated with heavy drinking, and it seemed logical to believe that alcohol was responsible.

We now know that cirrhosis can occur in people who never have consumed much alcohol—even in teetotalers. Rather, faulty nutrition now appears to be the essential cause. Its frequency among hard drinkers is a consequence of the fact that so often a hard drinker does not eat properly. The alcohol can cause gastritis, loss of appetite and disinterest in proper meals.

The alcohol provides calories, but it doesn't provide other necessities, such as protein and vitamins. The B-complex vitamins become so depleted that injections of them are very frequently given to hard drinkers when they at last start collapsing after a spree.

To be sure, the excessive accumulation of the intermediate products of alcohol metabolism as aldehydes can be toxic to the liver cells, but adequate diet tends to prevent changes from this.

More often than I like to contemplate, this question comes: "What can be done to cure cirrhosis of the liver?"

The unhappy answer is: Nothing. This is not a curable disease. Once it has occurred, it is there to stay. It is an actual and permanent change in the texture of the liver, and such cells as have been rendered inactive will stay that way.

The treatment of cirrhosis, as distinguished from cure, is to stop the process from going farther. Proper diet, not medicine, is the essential. And proper diet, not pills, is the best thing we can possibly adopt to keep the liver healthy. Alcohol should be stopped completely.

Another threat to the liver is fatty infiltration—fat particles invading and clogging the liver. Here again diet is the preventive. Obesity is harmful in many ways, and this is one.

There are some less common liver diseases, among them the formation of cysts from parasites, hemochromatosis (iron storage disease) and so on. Like any other part of the body, the liver can be attacked by cancer, which often spreads to it from some other part of the body.

But all of these are specialized and difficult problems, and since this book is a health book, not a disease book, let's stick to our

topic. Properly balanced diet, avoidance of obesity and avoidance of poisoning by excessive alcohol are by far the best ways to
assure a healthy liver. Then just let the liver go its way.

JAUNDICE AND WHAT IT REALLY IS

Quite a few people think jaundice is a disease. It isn't. Here's
a letter from a young woman who thought it was:

> Dear Doctor:
>
> What causes jaundice, and what is the cure for it? How
> serious is it? Can you catch it from someone who has a bad
> case of it? Even his eyes are very yellow.

Jaundice may involve either the liver, or the gall bladder, or
both—but it is a symptom. It is not a disease in itself.

The liver, remember, manufactures bile, a brownish or yellow-
green fluid that is intimately bound up with the process of digestion. The bile, bitter to the taste but extremely useful, contains
both bile salts and pigments (coloring matter).

The bile salts are absorbed through the intestine, to be returned
to the liver and used over again. The brownish or yellowish pigments are discharged from the body, accounting for the color of
the feces. This colored material, as a matter of fact, is the used-up
remnant of red blood cells that have served their purpose and
have been replaced by new ones.

If for some reason this yellow pigment cannot be discharged
from the body, it will gradually spread through the body. That is
the explanation of "yellow jaundice." The skin becomes tinged,
and often the whites of the eyes may be one of the first places to
show the color.

These pigments may be trapped in the body either because the
liver is affected in such a way that it cannot turn them into part
of the bile, or because, even though the liver may be able to do
that part of the task, it is unable to discharge the bile into its
normal course.

A disease occasionally seen in infants involves jaundice as an
outstanding symptom. In that case, the red cells being destroyed

at an excessive rate, so there is more pigment than the little body can get rid of.

Anyway, the liver produces bile constantly, some of it going directly to the duodenum, some of it going to the gall bladder, which is a reservoir for storage of the bile until (after we have eaten) we need a considerable amount.

From the gall bladder, the bile reaches the duodenum, or start of the small intestine, by flowing through a duct into the common duct, which also carries the bile directly from the liver.

Most cases of jaundice, therefore, result either from hepatitis, in which inflammation prevents the liver from operating correctly, or from blockage of the common bile duct.

This second situation may result from a gallstone working its way out of the gall bladder and becoming lodged in the common duct. This will be a painful matter immediately, and you will have no question as to whether to call the doctor. Or the duct may become blocked by a growth, in which case it may be painless but nevertheless urgently requires medical attention.

DISSOLVE GALLSTONES? No!

There are various diseases of the gall bladder but gallstones are by far at the top of the list.

Since bile carries concentrated solids (the bile salts and pigment) some of them can crystallize into "stones"; these may grow in size. There may be a single large stone in the gall bladder, or several. Or there may be many small ones called "sand" or "gravel."

Little ones may get into the duct and be carried through, perhaps causing colic or pain as they go, depending on size. Slightly larger ones will hurt more—and one that becomes firmly stuck in the duct can be exquisitely painful.

Too large a stone can't even begin passage and so must remain in the gall bladder. The possessor of it may not even be aware of its presence or may learn of it because other symptoms lead the doctor to have the gall bladder X-rayed.

It is then par for the course to ask how to get rid of the stones, sand or gravel. A typical inquiry:

Dear Doctor:

Isn't there something that will dissolve the stones? I do not wish to have an operation, but my doctor says he does not consider it safe to leave the stones.

Best way I've heard the answer put is this: There isn't any way to dissolve gallstones without dissolving the patient, too. That's the way it is, and we'll just have to put up with it. Facts are facts. True, efforts are being made to find a means of dissolving gallstones, but to date none are of practical value.

Neither is there any particular way of preventing gallstones except by certain rules of good health. Infections predispose to stone formation, and avoiding (or ending, as readily as possible) general infections is a good rule of health, quite apart from whatever direct discomfort or damage the infection may be causing.

Cholesterol also is a part of the chemical substance of gallstones, so abnormally high cholesterol levels may predispose a person to gallstone formation. Stasis (or extreme sluggishness), as in pregnancy, can be a factor.

There you have the principal known factors, and I think will agree that avoidance of gallstones is simply to be regarded as one more good reason for healthful living. There aren't any magic formulas for preventing stones.

Blocking of the common duct and the attendant pain is not the only good reason for getting rid of stones. Their continued presence can irritate the tissues and lead to infections and even to necrosis. Cancer occurs in some cases where gallstones have been allowed to remain.

The patient's age and physical condition, the degree of symptoms, the condition of the stones (quantity and length of time they have been there) are some of the elements which influence the decision. It is a matter of clinical judgment. If your doctor tells you the gall bladder ought to come out, my advice is to do as he says.

THE UNHEEDED CALL FOR "A DIET"

There are two inquiries which outnumber all others concerning the aftermath of a gall bladder operation. Here is a sample of each:

> Please send me a diet to be followed after a gall bladder operation. My doctor said I should be careful about my eating, but didn't give me a diet. Friends have told me that I ought to be on a regular gall bladder diet.

The other frequent one:

> I keep having gas and stomach distress even though I have had my gall bladder out—the doctor said it had a lot of gravel. I thought that my troubles would stop after having the operation, but I still have a great deal of discomfort. What can I do for relief?

Contrary to popular belief, no "gall bladder diet" is either necessary or useful. Many patients are able to continue eating exactly as they did before. Others may have to be a little careful in some respects, but no rigid or special diet is needed.

Keep in mind that the gall bladder wasn't a source of bile. It was just a storage place. The liver keeps right on making the same amount of bile after the removal. The difference is that all of it flows directly to the intestine, instead of having some of it saved up to be released when an extra amount is needed.

Since the bile is of particular importance in digesting fats, it may be advisable to limit the amount of fat consumed at any one meal. That doesn't mean you can't have any fat. You can have all you need for health. You just may have to avoid getting too much at once—so your eating habits clearly will have a lot to do with whether you have to change at all. Some do, some don't.

As to dyspepsia after the operation—it turns out that most victims will prove to have some other gastrointestinal disturbance. Irritable stomach or colon, ulcers or, indeed, just about any of the troubles we discussed in the chapter on digestion can be involved. Having the gall bladder out doesn't affect *them*.

PANCREAS—TOO MUCH OR TOO LITTLE?

The pancreas, a fairly close neighbor of the liver, is a well-protected organ, not particularly subject to injury but of considerable significance if it gets out of adjustment.

Its two main purposes are the production of enzymes needed for digestion and the production of insulin, which is required for the utilization of sugar by the system.

If not enough insulin is produced, sugar cannot be put to use and too much accumulates in the blood. Some of it "spills over" and can be detected in the urine.

When that happens, we call it diabetes mellitus, or "sugar diabetes."

In the opposite direction, the pancreas may produce too much insulin (a tumor being the likely cause of this) and sugar is used too rapidly. (This is immensely less common than diabetes.)

Then the trouble is "low blood sugar." A feeling of faintness and suddenly "being starved," weakness, tremors, nervousness, breathlessness and even brief blackouts are among the consequences.

Let me emphasize that this is far from the only cause of low blood sugar, or hypoglycemia. But it is the one that intimately involves the pancreas.

The larger aspect, by far, is diabetes, which numbers several million sufferers in the United States, and perhaps as many more who don't yet know that the disease is starting to affect them.

It is one of the health problems that is on the increase, while so many others are being prevented, suppressed or limited.

There's a reason. Until the 1920's, severe diabetes was quickly fatal. The victim, since he could not make use of sugar (starches, proteins and other foods are converted wholly or in part into sugar by the body), wasted away—actually starved—in spite of what he ate. Yet at the same time he dared not eat too much because the excess sugar in his system was accumulating as a direct threat to his life, too. A terrible and agonizing way to die? Yes, indeed.

Then came insulin. Overnight, people who were doomed suddenly had a new lease on life. With injections of sufficient insulin to compensate for the deficiency of the pancreas, their sugar utilization could be restored to normal balance.

If this balance is kept stable, there is no reason why a diabetic cannot live out a normal life span. A word of caution here: I am not saying that it is always easy to maintain this balance. There are what we call "brittle diabetics," who have to be watched closely to be sure that the balance is not upset. A little extra food, or a little less exercise to use up the sugar or an infection (even a minor cold or such), and sugar in the blood may start to rise.

Contrariwise, too little food, and more exertion and tension than usual may result in an excess of insulin, leading to an insulin reaction in which the patient may look as though he has had too much to drink and in short order may collapse.

When one of these attacks is coming on, a couple of pieces of candy, some fruit juice or pop can be enough to restore the balance for the critical moment, and the patient can be guided back to normal balance quickly. But suppose nobody realizes what is happening or what he needs? It can become a tragedy.

Diabetes cannot be taken lightly. Most patients can, if they follow instructions, do pretty much as they please about everything else. But if they disobey the rules, or if the "brittle" patients are unlucky, it can be disastrous. That's the kind of disease it is.

I've strayed, deliberately, from the point I was going to make. Diabetes, except very mild cases, used to be deadly. Now it is not, if reasonable care is taken.

It used to be that the victims who developed diabetes early in life died before they had time to raise families. Died—or were obviously too ill. The disease has a strong hereditary aspect. The victims of severe cases did not pass the trait along by having children.

Today the same kind of people with severe cases not only can have children but can live to bring them up. So there is more diabetes—but we can do so very much more about it. To my way of thinking, the net result is a great gain. But we *do* have more diabetics than we used to, and this trend will continue.

What Can We Do about Diabetes?

The exact cause of diabetes is not known. It isn't a germ, evidently. Heredity is a large factor, but it does not seem to be the whole story. While the diabetic must not eat more than a modest amount of sugar, because he can't handle it, and must keep his total food intake within reason because other foods translate into sugar, it does not appear that eating sugar has any bearing, in advance, on the development of diabetes. That is, eating sugar doesn't lead to "sugar diabetes."

On the other hand, obesity does. The overweight person is a prime candidate for diabetes. A slim person may become diabetic, true, but the preponderance is the other way. A tremendous majority of diabetics are people who have allowed themselves to become fat. Or at least overweight.

As for heredity, the risk rises geometrically. Therefore, if one parent comes from a family that has a history of diabetes, the risk of having children with diabetes isn't half as great, but instead is about one fourth as great as if both parents carry the trait. This isn't an exact mathematic formula, of course. Two people, both from strongly diabetic families, will be more likely to have diabetic children than two from mildly diabetic forebears. But the tendency is there.

It's a second thing we can do as a preventive, though. First, we can keep our weight normal. Second, we can do the best we can to avoid marriages when diabetes is known to exist in both families.

Third, we can take simple precautions to detect the disease as early as possible. The sooner it is recognized, the sooner it can be controlled and the less danger there is of drastic harm from it. The case that continues, uncontrolled, carries the risk of poor healing of wounds, blindness and other threats.

Each year the American Diabetes Association (and most of the physicians in the country) support Diabetes Week, during which people are urged to have simple urine tests. This is the best way of economically detecting cases. A single blood sugar test taken two hours after an average meal is a better detection tool. A sugar tolerance test can give even more precise information in suspicious cases.

I urge everyone to have a diabetes test periodically, particularly if he is overweight or has diabetes in his family. If you don't do so, at least keep in mind some of the signs of the disease: Excessive thirst, frequent urination, itching not readily ascribed to some other cause.

Frequent miscarriages or stillbirths, or having large babies (above 8 pounds) is another highly suspicious sign.

USE OF "DIABETES PILLS"

Are the so-called "diabetes pills" effective? Yes, in the right cases.

When diabetes starts in childhood or youth, it is virtually a fixed rule that insulin will be mandatory.

In the older person, and particularly when the case is light and is caught early, the pills often work very well. Sometimes losing some weight and then observing a careful diet is sufficient without further medication—although the patient should be careful to have his case checked regularly, perhaps each 6 months as long as things go smoothly. In other cases, a combination of the pills plus insulin is preferable.

The pills are not insulin. If we took insulin by mouth, it would be digested and no longer be insulin. In some adults the pancreas may be producing enough insulin, but the insulin's action is blocked by some vague factor not thoroughly understood. One theory is that the pills promote a greater release of insulin from the units or "islets" in the pancreas.

SOME OTHER INTERNAL ORGANS

The appendix we have already discussed. Another organ, the spleen, becomes of occasional interest. Its purposes in the body are not completely understood, but it plays a part both in the creation of some blood constituents and apparently, when the time comes, the destruction of others. It appears to be helpful as a storage area for blood and, for example, white cells, projecting them into the blood stream as needed.

In countries where malaria is rampant, the spleen often becomes considerably enlarged and sometimes can be ruptured rather easily. This is not a frequent problem in the United States, however, and probably the greatest element of danger is a serious accident that ruptures, tears or punctures the spleen.

Bleeding is profuse and an imminent threat to life. Since the tissue is soft, surgical repair is rarely possible. Fortunately, since the spleen is not an absolute necessity, it can be removed entirely, and the blood vessels connecting with it can be closed off. The lymph nodes enlarge afterward to compensate for some of the spleen's responsibilities; other organs share the rest.

Moving down in the abdominal cavity, we come to other organs that, for our own protection, we most certainly should understand. They are: kidneys, bladder, prostate and related organs.

The purpose of the kidneys is removal of wastes from the blood, as explained in Chapter V. The wastes are then discharged (as urine) into the bladder and finally leave the body through the urethra.

With healthy kidneys, as with the liver, "kidney pills" are of no service. If the kidneys are diseased, more specific treatment is necessary. However, the fiction that back pain, particularly low in the back, is a sign of "kidney trouble" perhaps fosters the reliance on pills. True, there may at times be some pain in the kidney region but it isn't in the lower back. In the majority of cases pain is of scant diagnostic use, and many cases of serious kidney disease develop without pain. There are, however, other effective methods of knowing the condition of the kidneys.

Any shutting off of the removal of poisons leads quickly to uremic poisoning; blockage of the flow below the kidneys must be promptly relieved not only for that reason but because the backing up of pressure can damage the kidneys themselves. Such an acute condition, however, is bound to be painful and will not permit the patient to postpone treatment.

The essential dangers are infection (pyelonephritis) of one kind or another attacking the kidneys and inflammation (glomerulonephritis or Bright's disease) leading to scarring and inactivating some of the millions of tiny "filter" units which make up the kidneys. Damage may also result from infections elsewhere that do not actually infect the kidney tissues themselves.

Study of urine specimens is one of the most useful diagnostic methods. It involves chiefly a search for pus, blood, dead cells and albumin (although in the case of this last, it can occur without necessarily indicating anything wrong).

Everyone should maintain a fixed rule of having prompt medical attention at any sign of blood or pus in the urine. Even amounts of blood too small to be recognized by a pink tinge can be indicative, so we can well modify the rule to say that examination is called for if the urine has a cloudy appearance, or if there is any marked change in urinary habits.

It should not be felt that any of these signs have to mean kidney disease. Many times the trouble will be in the bladder. That, too, demands prompt attention. One of the dangers, of course, is cancer, which can grow quite rapidly in the bladder. However, if treated immediately, when the first sign is noticed, it has a very high rate of cure.

HANDLING OF KIDNEY STONES

Kidney stones, unlike gallstones, often can be treated, to some degree at least, medically. If the stone is large, its removal generally must be by surgery, but smaller stones may be passed with the urine.

Chemically, these stones may be urates, oxalates or phosphates, and for each a different type of medication should be used to neutralize the chemicals that cause the stones. In addition, the patient must drink large quantities of liquids. If the urine is kept dilute, the chemicals are less likely to crystallize into "stones." If you have been bothered with stones, you have one of the simplest of all methods of preventive medicine—drink lots of water!

The so-called floating kidney upsets some people because they don't know what it means. The kidneys are surrounded by fat and loose tissues which cushion them against shock. If the kidney moves more than an average amount, it is a "floating kidney." It may be corrected surgically if necessary, but generally such a kidney is left alone unless it causes distress of some sort. The possibility of a ureter (duct from kidney to bladder) becoming kinked is probably the principal harm that can come from a floating kidney, but in the majority of cases no harm results from a kidney having a little extra room in which to move around.

The prolapsed or "fallen" bladder is in much the same category. The condition is the result of stretching or loosening (often caused by childbirth) the tissues which support it. If it isn't troublesome, usual practice is to let it alone.

Depending on the degree of displacement, incomplete voiding and puddling of urine may occur, thus setting up a natural breeding place for bacteria and thus fostering infection (cystitis). Plastic surgery can be done on the supporting tissues, restoring the bladder to suitable position.

In men, usually as they get on in years, trouble with the prostate becomes rather common. This organ, part muscle and part gland, is more or less doughnut-shaped and surrounds the urethra. If it becomes inflamed and swollen, it greatly reduces the force and volume of the flow of urine—if you recall, a few paragraphs back we suggested a change in urinary habits as one sign deserving medical attention. This is one application of the rule.

Treatment will have to be selected on the basis of the individual case, but when surgical removal is proposed, the safe course is to have it done. The reason? The prostate is one of the spots in which cancer tends to start. Since the prostate is so located as to permit access to it, cure of such cancers offers a good rate of success. The rule remains: Find it early, remove it early before it has a chance to spread and you may well be rid of it entirely. Procrastinate and you are in grave danger.

RECTAL TROUBLES AND HEMORRHOIDS

Here is a typical letter on this topic:

> Dear Doctor:
>
> I am very much bothered by hemorrhoids or "piles." I have used a number of remedies that were advertised and got relief from them but it was only temporary.
>
> I have been advised to have surgery but would like to avoid that. Some friends have told me about a clinic in _____ which guarantees that they can be cured without surgery. Can you give me some information about this method?

Well, hemorrhoids are nothing more nor less than varicose veins in the rectum. It would be obvious to all of us that salves wouldn't be the answer to varicose veins in the legs. In the case of hemorrhoids we are thrown of the trail of logic by the difference in terms.

Further, the hemorrhoids are so located as to be irritated. Itching and burning result. Salves or suppositories can ease this, but without doing anything to correct the underlying trouble, the swollen veins.

It sometimes is possible to shrivel small ones by electrocoagulation, but this is quite impractical when the veins are large. Injection procedure may also be effective in disposing of small hemorrhoids. Shopping around for "guaranteed" methods of treatment "without surgery" is a waste of time and money and pointless. Your own doctor (or the proctologist to whom he sends you) can tell you whether surgery is needed or some other treatment gives any promise. Your condition is what decides it, not a promise that you can avoid surgery.

Granted, removal of hemorrhoids is not the most pleasant experience in the world. You'll have several miserable days after it, but it is the route to permanent relief. There are two things you should keep in mind. One is to avoid constipation—that is covered under Maxim No. 7. The other is to go back to the doctor afterward if he finds dilation to be advisable. This, too, isn't pleasant, and some patients just don't go back when they are told to do so. However, it needn't be repeated many times, and it is good insurance against scar tissue preventing proper bowel action, with the threat of constipation and ultimate risk of the formation of more hemorrhoids. A certain amount of discomfort from the dilation is a good investment in future health and comfort.

Another very common complaint is pruritus—just a fancy term for itching. In this case it is pruritus ani, or itching of the anus.* It may be from hemorrhoids. Again, it may not. It is quite possible that some sort of allergy can be at work, but this is not easy to track down.

One method which I have found to be effective in a good many cases is quite simple. First, be scrupulously clean. By that I mean washing the area after bowel action, then drying it. And finally

---

* See Chapter 10 for a more general discussion of pruritus.

place a small pledget of absorbent cotton so that the area will be kept dry. This is not a substitute for having treatment for hemorrhoids, remember, but for itching.

If this fails, your doctor may find a clue pointing to some other means of allaying the itching.

13

FOR WOMEN ONLY

MAXIM 13 *Facts, not fables, will keep you safe from the "women's diseases." They aren't as mysterious as they have been made to seem.*

A young woman in college casually mentioned that she had gone to the doctor for a pelvic examination. There was nothing wrong, it turned out—just a clean bill of health.

The girl's mother, however, was surprised.

Daughter simply explained that she had read so much about feminine disorders that she decided to have a checkup.

I say good for her! The difference in viewpoint between mother and daughter was, perhaps, the difference in viewpoints between two generations. The older generation was taught to be reticent about all such things. The younger generation is learning that, while modesty remains a worthy characteristic, too much reticence does not make sense. It can be harmful. It can be dangerous. It can, in some instances, be downright deadly.

On the other hand, accepting the obvious fact that the female organs are part of the human body, and that every woman has them, and that they may get out of order and need checking and treatment from time to time, is only good sense.

Nature gave us our bodies. It is for us to take care of them.

The small child has no false modesty. The child will ask questions! It is the preceding generation which says, "Shush, we don't talk about such things."

The child in such cases is smarter than the parent.

In one family of my acquaintance, the phrase "family talk" solves any difficulties which arise. The children, now growing up, have been told, ever since they were old enough to understand, that some things are family talk and others are not. If they asked questions about their bodies (or about such things as the family's finances, or other personal matters!) they were told, "Here is the answer to your question, but remember, this is 'family talk.' We don't discuss it except among ourselves."

These youngsters are now growing up with the realization that they can ask about anything they want to. If it is something not to be talked about generally, they "keep the lip buttoned." They don't blurt out embarrassing remarks at the dinner table, but neither do they feel that there are certain questions which, for reasons unknown to them, they must not ask even in private.

It seems to me that this is the sane and healthful way to handle the matter. That college girl whom I mentioned has no false notions. She isn't going to blab about her pelvic condition over the dinner table, but she is going to have checkups at reasonable intervals and isn't going to suffer for years in silence if some painful or annoying or even dangerous condition threatens.

For only one example of what undue modesty can cause, I cannot forget a fine woman who died agonizingly of rectal cancer because she had been brought up "too modestly" to tell her doctor of the early symptoms. Any physician knows of similar cases. In that instance it was a matter of rectal bleeding which she should have reported to her doctor, but the principle is the same. If she had had vaginal bleeding, she would have been too modest to mention that.

I'm going to return to this aspect a little later in this chapter, but please keep in mind that while we rightly may not care to discuss the problems of the uterus in the living room nor want to tell all the neighbors what the doctor said we should do about that annoying discharge, we *do* tell our doctors. By doing so we cure these troubles instead of suffering in silence.

Where Questions Come From

It seems elementary, doesn't it, that as a girl reaches her teens, she should know how her body works. Too often we, as parents, don't tell her. And, pray, how else are girls to learn except by exchanging mutually mistaken information among school friends?

Admittedly most of us balk at the idea of sitting down and saying, "Now let's have a nice little talk about the birds and bees." Or the "facts of life," or whatever term we happen to think up. Besides, as a parent myself, I must admit that to adults the youngsters seem to grow up with such surprising speed. Most of us do not realize that the girl is becoming a woman—until all of a sudden she has done so, and it seems a little late to discuss the matters that we had been vaguely intending to tackle "when the right time came."

Occasionally I receive a letter from a puzzled mother asking how to go about presenting the information. They don't often ask me. I suppose they know that they aren't going to receive an answer that will be satisfactory. For, indeed, there isn't much I can say, at that point, except that launching into the subject with a teen-age daughter is likely to be embarrassing to both mother and daughter. The groundwork has to be prepared before that.

My advice, strange as it may seem at first glance, is to leave things to the daughter. Wait for her to ask the questions. She will. But now comes the important thing. Make it a rule never to evade or postpone a question!

This means starting with the questions of childhood. Don't say, "When you are older, you'll understand." Give a factual answer to the question, whatever it is. I don't suggest going into great detail. Anyway, the child doesn't want a complicated reply. She wants the briefest, simplest answer possible to the question she asked. As she learns that she can expect such answers—which are, after all, the kind of answers you automatically give to her questions about anything else—she will quite naturally keep on asking more questions as they occur to her.

Put off answering her early questions, and she won't ask the questions that occur to her later. Or she won't ask *you*.

Thus it is that for every question from a mother, I get many from daughters. One rather frequent one is simply:

"My friend and I are both 15, but have not started to have our period yet. A lot of friends started two years ago. What should we do? And what is the matter with us?"

Nothing is the matter with them, and there isn't anything to do except wait. Nature's ingenuity is breath-taking when you pause to consider how she establishes the cyclic changes that are so important. But Nature chooses her own timing. Menstruation begins somewhere between the ages of 11 and 16, the average being about 13½. Race, climate, rate of growth and any number of factors may be involved in the precise timing of the onset; much of the time we are unable to specify any particular cause. But it doesn't matter. When Nature is ready, that is the right time.

Incidentally, menstruation, while it is a signal that the child is becoming a woman, does not necessarily imply fertility. It can be two to three years, in some cases, before conception is possible.

There is another variation which causes considerable worry but doesn't mean anything. Taking another letter at random:

> Dear Doctor:
>
> I am nearly 15, and started menstruating about seven months ago. I had three periods and then they stopped.
>
> I absolutely know that I haven't done anything that I shouldn't, but one of my friends says that when you stop menstruating it is a sign that you are pregnant. I haven't dared say anything to my mother about this, but I am worried to death about it.

Of course she was worried about it. And I couldn't help thinking, also, that here was a perfect illustration of a young girl who *ought* to feel free to talk to her mother, but they hadn't established that kind of relationship. Frightened, she worried and finally wrote to me.

The menses may be quite irregular at first. With some girls, regularity may start and continue pretty much like clockwork, but it is more often the rule for the interval to be uncertain at first, and a lapse of several months is not unusual—all without indicating anything wrong.

Each girl gradually assumes her own pattern, and although the 28-day cycle is average, there is nothing to indicate that everyone has to be average. Regulation of the time is under control of hormones (See Chapter XII). A rise in estrogen (female sex hormone) of the ovaries causes a change in the lining of the uterus in order to prepare it to accept a fertilized ovum, should such an ovum (egg) arrive.

If fertilization has not occurred, further changes in hormone secretion cause the prepared membrane to slough off from the lining of the uterus. This is menstruation. Its purpose is not, as some suppose, intended to remove an unfertilized ovum, for the ovum is tiny, of cell size, and would need no such measures to remove it.

Not "Riddance of Poison"

The function of menstruation is not, as some of the ancients, and even some of the not-so-ancients, have believed, a "riddance of poison." It simply clears the way for a fresh preparation of the uterine lining in case, in the coming cycle, a fertilized ovum should be presented.

There are so many fables about menstruation that we could hardly list them all. There is the incorrect—and probably often harmful—expression that it is a woman's "sick time."

She isn't sick. She is perfectly normal, perfectly healthy. This every young woman should be brought up to realize. Otherwise, there may follow all sorts of incorrect beliefs. The commonest of these are the notions that menstruation should limit a woman's physical activities. This is not true, but from letters written to me I can say very definitely that such ideas are quite widespread.

One is: "My mother says I shouldn't wash my hair at this time, or take a bath or a shower. Why is this?" a girl asks.

There isn't any reason why she shouldn't—except a groundless fable that probably has been passed from mother to daughter for generations. Nobody seems to be able to explain what is supposed to be wrong with washing one's hair, or keeping clean in general; perhaps whoever started the fable didn't have any reason in mind, either.

Other young women want to know if it is true that they shouldn't dance, or play tennis or golf. The answer again is that no harm will come to them. In fact, it may even help them. Some very serious searching studies have been made among college women on the subject of menstruation and exercise. The one important finding was this, and it was very definite: The young women who regularly got plenty of exercise had very little if any trouble with cramps; those who got little exercise were the ones who complained of cramps in connection with menstruation. Nature didn't intend us to sit still too much of the time. Activity is normal and good for us.

It also is pretty much an axiom among physicians that the more nervous tension exists, the more complaints are bound to arise. The neurotic woman may become just about an invalid at this time, but not because of physical reasons so much as for psychological ones. She may subconsciously resent being a woman. (Who knows? If the same person were a man we might find resentment against *that!*) She may be responding to attitudes subtly implanted by her elders, accepting feelings and resentments that stem from something else. Some women, I regret to say, are brought up in the habit of using menstruation as a means of evading routine duties. This sort of thing starts, in my belief, with such things as telling a daughter that she should stay home from school because of the menstrual period.

By this I do not mean that menstrual discomfort cannot occur. It can—but in a minority of cases. Going a little farther back in the cycle, some women have a sharp pain when a follicle ruptures in the ovary, and the ovum emerges. The majority do not feel anything. This pain can be useful when one wishes to become pregnant and wants to know when the ovum has begun its trip through one of the Fallopian tubes and is ready for fertilization. Otherwise, it is an unasked pain and, in a few instances, can be decidedly uncomfortable.

It is quite general, however, for fluid to accumulate in the system for a few days before menstruation starts. Nature is storing fluids. There may be a sensation of bloating or heaviness for a couple of days, to be relieved when menstruation begins. Engorgement and tenderness of the breasts may be an accompaniment. Headache is sometimes another companion or, if not exactly a headache, perhaps a sensation of fullness and tension.

In a very few annoying cases, this accumulation of fluid can be a distressing problem. Since the word *fluid* translates into *water* for all practical purposes of weight, a few pints of fluid means a few pounds. So women who are watching their weight should remember this and not be misled by the temporary gain in weight at this time. It is just a certain amount of water that gathers in the system, then is lost again.

A Whole New Wardrobe?

Think what happens, however, if the amount is excessive, perhaps a dozen pints and hence a dozen pounds, more or less. One reader wrote to me:

> I gain so much that my clothes are uncomfortably tight, and some of my dresses are so tight I can't wear them at all. I am careful about my eating, but even this does not seem to help at all. I'm sure this is not normal. Is there any treatment that can correct this trouble? My clothes fit so badly that I do not want to go out of the house until I am back to my regular weight.

Not many women have such an extreme problem, but a few have even more difficulty. One modern classic concerned an employee of a hospital. It happened to be a hospital at which the research staff was making a study of this very problem. In this woman's case, she gained so much weight—which means fluid—that she had to have two wardrobes, one for ordinary wear and another, a couple of sizes larger, for the several days a month when she just could not wear her regular clothes. She now needs only one wardrobe.

Treatment varies. Use of diuretics (drugs to impel excretion of fluids) is one. Antispasmodic drugs, sedatives, tranquilizers and dilation of the cervix in extreme cases are other measures. This last is done of the theory that a small outlet in the cervix may retard release of fluids.

After the first pregnancy, this particular type of difficulty tends to subside, which is a happy circumstance.

Pregnancy, either directly or indirectly, solves a good many troubles. Painful, crampy menstruation becomes easier in many cases, for example.

More important, perhaps, is that a young woman who may have had little or no contact with a gynecologist finally does so because of becoming pregnant. She may be cared for by a general practitioner, or she may, as so many now do, have a specialist in obstetrics and gynecology.

More than a few then realize for the first time that most menstrual troubles can be alleviated if not relieved entirely, once the physician is told about the troubles. The doctor isn't a mind-reader, so don't suffer in silence!

PROBLEMS OF THE BREAST

Size may not be the most important problem concerning the breast, but I sometimes wonder if it isn't the question which preoccupies more women than any other. To tell the truth, when a new wave of letters comes sweeping at me, I get to wondering: Isn't there *anything* we can do to control this bustomania which gets so much encouragement from the movies and entertainment world, and sometimes advertising?

By the age of 14, high school girls are busy writing to me for advice on how to achieve bigger bust measurements. Some of them start fretting even younger than that. Likewise I'm getting the same kind of questions from women who are 20 or 25 years older. Isn't *anybody* satisfied with whatever endowment Nature provided?

Size of the breast is pretty much governed by two things: hormone control and deposition of fat—for the breast is largely composed of fatty tissues. The thin, small-framed foman is likely to have small breasts. The same is true of the woman with deficient ovarian or pituitary hormone secretions.

Despite the clamor, not to say insistence, that I offer some easy way to expanding the bustline, there isn't any easy answer. The best solution is to know what can be done with what is available. The high school girl who is thin as a rail because her growth has gone to height will find that the breasts will fill out as she puts on enough weight to catch up to her height.

The stoop-shouldered or slouchy girl, if we can only open her eyes, often learns that good posture will do wonders for her. If she will stand up straight and throw back her shoulders, it will make a lot more difference than she realizes. I suggest that such girls take a good analytical look at fashion photographs, for the professional models are usually thin, too, and anything but big-busted, but they know how to stand.

Many a young women is still filling out when she is in her twenties, sometimes pretty well along in the twenties, too. Pregnancy and nursing sometimes makes a difference, although there is no way to predict this.

If none of these works, the only answer is falsies, and since dresses are designed for average bustlines, I can't see any reason why a little padding isn't warranted. I have, however, had one or two worried letters to the effect that "I am to be married next month and Herbert doesn't know I wear falsies." If "Herbert" doesn't have at least an inkling by that time, I'd be rather surprised, and I don't think the girls need be too concerned. Besides, it may be, after all, that a bumper crop of bosom isn't necessarily of such universal appeal as is presumed. I, for one, can remember back to the days of the John Held, Jr. cartoons, when the goal of every girl was to be flat as a board, and they went to extremes to flatten the breast.

Don't ask me to explain the vagaries of fashion. I'm just a doctor! But creams, hormones, massage and home-grown ointments such as cocoa butter all are usually quite futile.

Don't think this is the only type of question, though. Numerous, although well outnumbered, are questions about what can be done about the too-large breast and the sagging breast.

For the former, it pretty generally comes down to a matter of obesity. "I just cannot get a brassière that fits me, and as a result I am always uncomfortable," one woman wrote. "What can I do to reduce it by a few inches? I am 5 feet 4 and weigh 180, and have always been on the husky side."

By "husky," I'm afraid she means that from childhood on she has been accustomed to eating too much, and it perhaps has never really crossed her mind that taking off 20 or 30 pounds might be the whole answer, not to mention improving her general health and life expectancy. The breast is one of the natural depositories for fat in women.

Although repeatedly asked, I still say, "No, I do not recommend plastic surgery to increase the bust." Inserting foreign substances into the body in this fashion does not strike me as a safe thing to do, especially in view of the nature of the tissues involved. Neither have I any great faith in the degree of improvement possible. Yes, we hear from time to time about the supposedly wonderful things being done along this line in Japan or some other distant place, but as Omar said, "Oh, the brave music of a *distant* drum." And the appealing promises of a *distant* experiment.

The overly large breasts, as I said, are generally a weight-reducing problem, not a surgical one. (Rarely is excessive glandular activity involved.

The pendulous and sagging breast, however, is another matter entirely. Many times it is a result of reducing drastically—after having been drastically overweight too long. If it is merely a matter of some flabbiness, appropriate brassières are the best answer, and the most economical, too.

Where the situation warrants, however, this is something which can be helped by plastic surgery. Good plastic surgery is not cheap. It must be done by a highly trained and skilled surgeon who knows exactly what he wants to accomplish and how to do it. If the case is severe enough to make the cost worthwhile, excellent results can be obtained.

However, as a matter of good health, rather than of cosmetic values, I suggest that we take care of our diets, our posture and such similar basic rules of health as I have outlined in earlier chapters and not get too engrossed in trying to make medicine and surgery change Nature's handiwork.

Health of the breasts reduces itself for the most part to some understanding of lumps. (Skin troubles, which occasionally may occur there as well as anywhere else, and such matters as the inverted nipple are obvious enough and will be taken care of routinely by your regular physician.)

A lump in the breast has become synonymous with breast cancer in the minds of most women. This is not true, but I am willing to let things stand as they are, because breast cancer is the most prevalent of all types of cancer among women, and a strong suspicion of any lump is a lifesaving characteristic.

A single, painless lump should be regarded with the greatest suspicion so far as cancer is concerned.

The one objection I might have to the lump-equals-cancer attitude is that sometimes it becomes so strong that a woman delays reporting such a lump because—well, as in this letter:

> Dear Doctor:
>
> I have noticed a lump in my left breast for some time, and it seems to be getting a little larger although I am not sure about it. I have put off going to the doctor because of the fear that it might be cancer. Now I am beginning to notice one in the right breast, too. . . .

My answer? It probably is *not* cancer, but the sooner we can get this woman to see her doctor, the sooner she is going to have some peace of mind, and that is important, as I look at things.

But when a woman postpones seeing her doctor "because it might be cancer," that is the exact opposite of the intended reaction.

Where *fear* delays having a potential cancer sign examined, the whole purpose of all these warnings is turned end for end. We defeat ourselves. For the lump that is reported as soon as it is noticed is the one that has the highest percentage of cure—if, indeed, it *is* cancer. The statistics on breast cancer are not very encouraging. In spite of all the warnings, all the information on breast cancer, mortality has not changed visibly for a decade or more. Fear, I am distressed to think, is costing as many lives as it is saving. Therefore I think there may be a valid point in my own argument that we should place more stress on the fact that perhaps only one lump in thirty or so means cancer.

Cystic mastitis (an enlargement of glands in the breast, due to hormone activity) is the largest cause of lumps in the breast.

There may be one lump, or there may be several. Usually there will be lumps in both breasts, not just one. The lumps may be associated with a yellowish or greenish discharge from the nipples.

The breasts will be, or may be, tender. Discomfort will fluctuate with the menstrual cycle.

I am reluctant to speculate on how many women have detected these cystic lumps and lived in abject terror until driven by sheer fright to tell their doctors. It must be many times the number who have actually had cancer, and many of even these have been successfully treated.

If only a single cyst occurs, it is often difficult to differentiate it from cancer by any test save biopsy. The answer? Removal of the cyst so that it can be sent to the laboratory for a definite diagnosis. This does *not* mean removal of the whole breast, as, unfortunately, many women fear. It means removal only of the cyst (or lump). That is a relatively simple procedure and not disfiguring. Better a cyst in the bottle than a cancer in the breast!

How to test yourself for a lump? Lie flat on your back. Raise one arm above your head. Then with the palm of the other hand, reach across and palpate the breast—in other words, rub the palm completely around the breast. Pinching with the fingers will lead you onto all sorts of false clues. Perfectly normal tissue will feel like a lump. If there is a real lump, the pressure of the palm will detect it.

Films, booklets and pamphlets issued by the American Cancer Society and other groups will give greater detail, but about two minutes of time or less, and remembering to use the flat of the hand, will give you the substance of the method.

THE WOMAN OF 30 OR MORE

Dear Doctor:

My doctor tells me that I have a fibroid tumor but he has recommended not doing anything about it. His expression was, "Let's not bother it unless it bothers you. We'll just keep an eye on it."

Will this turn into cancer? If not, how much trouble can it cause? Will it prevent pregnancy? What can I do about it?

Only a very few years ago this question (or letters like it) were more numerous than they are today. There is a growing understanding of what fibroid tumors (or "fibroids") are, and this is a good thing.

The uterus is made up of muscle and fibrous tissue. When tumors occur, they appear in the latter, the fibrous tissues. They are "fibroids."

There may be one, or several, or many—I believe the record in medical history is well over a hundred tumors in one patient. (The uterus was removed, and she enjoyed excellent health thereafter.)

These tumors as a rule are not malignant, but they should be watched, once discovered, lest one become malignant or, in fact, be malignant from the start. If there is no indication of malignancy (cancer) they may well be left alone so long as they cause no other difficulty. At menopause, they sometimes regress—become smaller and simply exist in harmless desuetude.

If the tumors develop on the inner wall of the uterus, they can cause irregular bleeding or excessive and prolonged menstrual flow. They *may*. They may not. They may prevent pregnancy or make it difficult. They may, at times, reach such a size as to be painful or otherwise a nuisance. If they occur on the outer wall of the uterus, they may cause no symptoms whatever.

Appearance of fibroids, depending on size and number, what if any difficulty they may be causing and whether they are increasing in size is a common cause for hysterectomy (removal of the uterus). Fibroids may be felt by pelvic examination, and any change can be noted. I cannot possibly give any general answer as to whether they should or should not be removed—none that the patient can use. But I can say this: Fibroids are anything but rare. Their behavior is well known. If your doctor advises you to ignore them, except for a routine periodic check, let it go at that. If he finds reason for removal, he will tell you that, too.

There is no special age at which fibroids appear, except for the generality that they are more likely during the long span of childbearing years and are less likely after the high hormonal activity has ceased with menopause.

Another problem of the after-30 time is endometriosis, which in simplified terms means that some of the uterine lining has escaped through the Fallopian tubes and become implanted elsewhere within the pelvic region. It is displaced tissue—but it still responds to the influence of the ovarian hormones, still tries to create a fresh covering membrane each month, and then slough it off, but without a way of getting rid of the slough.

The result can be anything from the development of painful menstruation to an apparent bladder or bowel difficulty. Until recently, removal of the ovaries was the preferred treatment, for with the ovaries gone, ovarian hormones no longer were present to cause the cyclic changes. Today, hormones to prevent ovulation (and hence menstruation) are being used with success. This is the same type of drug used to prevent conception.

WHAT DOES HYSTERECTOMY MEAN?

Hysterectomy is one of those words that "everyone understands," but there are all sorts of incorrect notions about it—which, of course, is true of a good many others.

Specifically, it means surgical removal of the uterus (womb). These days this usually includes removal of the cervix, or neck of the uterus. It may or may not involve removal of one or both of the Fallopian tubes, and one or both of the ovaries.

What is the essential result of hysterectomy, aside from removal of some harmful or dangerous condition? Why, the result is that the patient no longer can have children, and that is about the sum total of the difference. Without the uterus, there no longer is a place for a fertilized ovum to be nurtured.

Yet all sorts of fictions have grown up, asserting that more basic changes occur. For a sample of some of the scare stories, as well as a couple of very pointed questions, take this letter from a "Mrs. D."

> Dear Doctor:
>
> At the age of 40 I had a complete hysterectomy, and have been a nervous wreck ever since. Do you ever get completely over an operation like this? Do you get over it faster when they leave an ovary or part of one? What is the purpose of that? I am getting medication for hot flashes and dizziness.

First off, the operation itself is no more dangerous than any of the many varieties of major surgery with which we are all familiar. It is a major operation, to be sure, and no surgery is to be taken lightly or casually. It is performed when there is a need for it, but it is not something to dread when it *is* needed. Time in the hospital will usually be about two weeks, and the patient, once home again, will resume full activity gradually.

We don't go around telling our friends that having the gall bladder removed, or the appendix, or a thyroid operation or even such serious things as heart surgery or removal of a lung is going to make a drastic change in their lives. Rather, we are happy when our friends have had their operations and are back on their feet, getting back to normal life again.

But the hysterectomy? Oh, no! We get the word around that there is something special about it, and the result is an ingrained feeling like Mrs. D's, as portrayed in her letter.

"Do you ever get completely over an operation like that?"

The right answer is a plain "Yes" (except that childbearing is ended).

Removal of the uterus has, except for the elimination of pregnancy, no effect whatsoever on femininity, sex life and activity or anything else. Those are the physical facts. Such emotional facets as may be instigated from hearing scare stories are quite another matter. If a woman has been taught that hysterectomy is going to make sweeping and drastic changes, she will have difficulty *not* letting her subconscious beliefs create imaginary troubles for her in later life. So it's important, don't you think, to implant sensible ideas and not old wives' tales.

There is just one aspect of hysterectomy that can be of very considerable importance, quite apart from the trauma of any surgery. That is removal of the ovaries. That brings us to a matter of very legitimate and real interest to every woman: menopause.

THE MEANING OF MENOPAUSE

Menopause, of course, means the end of the childbearing stage of a woman's life. It is an emotional experience of no small dimensions, even though the woman may never have had any children and, for that matter, may never have wanted any. It is still an important milestone in her life.

Please keep in mind that we have not finished answering Mrs. D.'s letter. She said that she had had a complete hysterectomy, meaning that tubes and ovaries as well as the uterus were removed.

The ovaries are the organs of importance now. The ovaries are endocrine glands. Besides releasing an ovum once a month for something like 30 years or so, the ovaries also secrete hormones into the system.

At menopause, the ovaries cease their activity. This occurs as a rule in the forties, and 45 is a fair enough average. It may be a few years earlier or a few years later, but it is rare past the age of 50, and 52 is the latest age at which there is any authentic record of a woman having a baby.

Some women encounter menopause at a little past 40, which keeps things within the bounds of normal averages. In some few instances involving some upset of the usual health and hormone balance, menopause may occur before 40, but this, too, is rare.

Thus menopause is almost always a matter of the early, late or middle forties. The ovaries gradually cease their activities, and this also means a cessation of menstruation.

This is something of a hit-or-miss affair. It does not happen all at once. Menstrual periods become irregular. One or more may be missed, after which one or more will occur. That is, one month an ovum will be released and will be followed by a menstrual flow to slough off the uterine lining. The next month there may be no ovum, no sloughing.

I must say that things are not quite as simple as I have made them out to be, because I am trying to give a general picture of what happens, and the whole complicated pattern of ovum-hormones-menstruation is not that easy. But please excuse me from exposing you to about two books full of highly technical talk —which would be the alternative.

Since menopause results from the retirement of the ovaries from activity, it is clear that surgical removal of the ovaries will do the same thing. This is called "surgical menopause." It is a more abrupt change, but aside from that the consequences are alike. This includes the fact that symptoms will vary widely in degree from one woman to another. Some have scant complaint. Others find the symptoms most annoying.

The principal symptom is hot flashes, sudden flashes of a feeling of heat and flushing of the skin which come without warning. Many feel as though they are blushing deeply; it can be noticeable to someone watching closely, but is not as apparent as the patient thinks it is. The feeling of warmth is no illusion, however. It is real, and an equally sudden burst of perspiration can accompany it.

Nervousness, tension and their manifestations are other consequences—yet for all the unpleasantness that can at times occur, it is not a harmful or dangerous matter. It is, remember, a natural occurrence, a phase of life. It may be as temporarily upsetting as adolescence. Many a parent of a teen-ager will testify that *that* can be a period of uneasy adjustment, too!

Where menopausal symptoms are severe, periodic administration of estrogenic hormones is helpful, holding the endocrine balance closer to its original level while the patient adjusts to the new level. A great many women do not require this—after all, over the centuries they had to get along without such treatment.

Neither should the patient ever get the idea that the use of hormones should be permanent. It is for the transition only. Their use ordinarily is for a matter of 6 months or a year. I do not recommend their use indefinitely.

How Long Does It Last?

One of the unanswerable questions about the menopause is duration of this transitional stage. How long does it take a growing-up teen-ager to get past the difficult stage? In either case, if it happens to be a particularly tense transition, it may last 6 months or a year—but seem like a century to those concerned.

Once ovarian activity has entirely ceased, then childbearing is permanently ended, of course, but the discomforts of the transition do *not* last forever. This is a fact which some women forget. As witness this:

Dear Doctor:

I have been having menopause symptoms for 9 years now, and still have hot flashes in spite of taking hormones. Isn't there anything else that can be done for this? I don't see how I can stand this for the rest of my life.

This is an abnormal situation, and the woman deserves some careful medical checking. When hot flashes continue years beyond the normal time it is no longer safe or sensible to keep blaming the menopause. Something else is happening. Careful study of the thyroid may afford a useful clue in a case such as this.

Menopause generally is too much used as a handy "waste basket" into which to toss any old symptom that happens along. It should not be forgotten, although it too often is, that other conditions can be developing at the same time. At the age of 45 or 50 we are well launched into what we vaguely call "the middle years." After half a century of wear and tear, our organs may at times be getting cranky. We don't have and shouldn't expect to have the energy, stamina and resilience of youth.

It is, in short, the time at which we should already have begun paying stricter attention to our health, and that is why it isn't safe to attribute every unexplained symptom to "the change of life."

One of the great fictions of yesteryear, now happily waning but not entirely gone, was the belief that menopause could cause mental illness. Irritability, yes, but not mental illness. Sometimes emotional illness may manifest itself at that time of life. It can strike at any age. But menopause doesn't cause it.

Another frequent question, probably the most frequent of all, is the possibility of pregnancy. "Dear Doctor: I have not had a period for a year and a half. Can I still become pregnant?" This inquiry, with variations in the timetable, keeps coming week after week, year after year. Or: "I am 51. Am I safe from pregnancy?"

The only way to answer it is by the general rule familiar to every doctor: The possibility of pregnancy can be considered past when one year has gone by since the last period. It is not a matter of age. It is a question of when no ovum can be present for fertilization.

For practical purposes, pregnancy is highly unlikely somewhat sooner than is stated in the above rule-of-thumb, but waiting a year gives a substantial margin of safety. There is no sharp, definable cutoff point. As menstruation becomes irregular at the beginning of menopause, there may be months during which pregnancy cannot occur, others during which it can—although as we move up in the age-40 bracket, there is gradually less chance of pregnancy.

As to the so-called "menopause baby," this is a baby conceived somewhere around the menopause age. There is no capricious flare-up of fertility. There is, instead, a gradual decline. But there is a considerable variance in the age at which menopause comes to different women, just as there is wide difference in fertility.

Tying the Fallopian Tubes

Tying the Fallopian tubes, thus shutting off the route by which the ovum would move from ovary to uterus, is a fairly simple procedure and is used as a means of preventing conception.

It prevents pregnancy but has no other physiological effect. The ovaries continue their usual secretion of hormones, and the resultant process of menstruation continues.

Because it sounds so simple (I presume) I am quite frequently asked about the advisability of having it done. I do not consider it to be within my province to try to tell people what they should decide for themselves, but I do urge the greatest thought before taking this step.

Why? Because I receive nearly as many letters from other readers who have had this procedure performed in the past and now want to know, "Can I have the tubes restored to their former condition?" They have, sometimes, read of such restorative operations in Baltimore or elsewhere.

True, it has been accomplished, but restoring is many times more difficult than the original tying, and sometimes the effort does not succeed at all.

In passing, a comparable operation, the vasectomy, is sometimes performed on men. This interrupts the duct through which the male sperm must pass. This, too, is moderately simple surgery but is just as serious a decision.

From too many letters from disappointed people I have learned that time and circumstances can lead us to change our minds drastically. I am, for this reason, unwilling to recommend these operations except for the most compelling reasons, and I *never* even discuss them without this proviso: Do not consider them unless you are content, and will always be content, that they be permanent. Never gamble that you can "have things changed back again" if you change your mind. There is too high a probability that you can't.

Before we leave the matter of surgery, let's go back to a point which I skipped over rather lightly, the question of what happens if the ovaries are or are not removed. When, in weighing the extent of a hysterectomy, one has to decide whether to remove or preserve the ovaries, or one of the two ovaries, the woman's age becomes important. If she is in her forties or almost there, removal of the ovaries advances the menopause by only a relatively short time.

On the other hand, if the woman is in her thirties or is younger, every reasonable effort is made to preserve at least one ovary. The purpose may be more psychological than physical, but psychological impact is no small matter.

Removal of the ovaries does not "make a woman old." Neither does it in any way affect or interfere with her sexual activity—and this is equally true of the menopause. All the same, from the psychological approach, it is preferable that she experience menopause at about the age originally intended by Nature. If it seems that I harp consistently on the idea of using the science of medicine as an assistant to Nature, rather than as a means of trying to achieve something better than Nature intended, that is correct. That *is* my attitude. Medicine is the handmaiden, not the queen.

Removal of the ovaries? When they are diseased or impaired (and not as Nature intended), then remove them whenever the need is plain.

A "We Don't Talk About It" Topic

In recent years we have discarded a lot of the old taboos. Quite rightly, we don't quibble about saying that we are going to have a baby instead of hinting delicately about a "blessed event." Not, of course, that a baby isn't a blessed visitor!

We talk frankly enough about most of the operations we have, except perhaps the hemorrhoidectomy, and that isn't always off limits.

But one very widespread problem still remains in the category of "we don't talk about it." This is the vaginal discharge. Well, it ought to be talked about, because it affects a great many women, and because nobody else ever seems to mention it, most of them don't tell their doctors until they can't keep quiet any longer. They thus suffer along, sometimes for a good many years, with something that should be treated early and easily.

The vagina is lined with mucous membranes containing appropriate small glands. The membrane is moist, and there may be a slight discharge normally. Invariably there will be a slight increase at mid-cycle, coinciding with ovulation.

When a discharge is heavy and persistent, it is an indication of something wrong. It is not natural, and hence should be reported and treated.

One teen-ager wrote to me, just before I began this chapter:

> Dear Doctor:
>
> I am 15 and have been having this discharge that stains my panties. I asked my mother about it, and she said to never mind it because it would go away and didn't mean anything. It just keeps on, and I wanted to write to you and ask you.

She added a P.S. to her letter: "I am sure it can't be a venereal disease because I have never done anything that would lead to that."

There are several causes of such discharges, all of them amounting to some sort of irritation. Commonest of all causes for heavy discharge is trichomoniasis, or the presence of a microorganism of the protozoon family, trichomonas vaginalis. This parasite, which for whatever reason, flourishes in the vagina, causes a heavy, yellowish and often odorous discharge. How it starts is not clear. One thought is that wearing tight panties and slacks may have some effect, but the "how" and "wherefore" remain to be discovered.

The perfectly "good" girl can acquire this sort of trouble. The single as well as the married can be victims. Neither age nor youth is a guaranteed protection. Like influenza or mumps, it can happen to anybody! But unlike influenza or mumps, once it gets started, it doesn't cease by itself.

In heavy attacks of trichomoniasis (and doubtless in lighter cases, too) a wife may infect her husband. It doesn't annoy him as it does her. But after she has been treated to get rid of the trouble, she can then be reinfected by her husband.

Yeast infections also can irritate the vagina. So can organisms of the monilial (fungus) family. They are found more frequently in women with diabetes, or women in menopause.

Briefly, a variety of microscopic organisms can invade the vagina, cause irritation (vaginitis) and result in a chronic discharge.

It is, obviously, true that more savage infections also will cause discharges. Infection of the tubes or other organs may be present. There may be "erosion of the cervix," meaning some sort of infection is causing ulceration of that area; a discharge is to be expected along with it.

Acute gonorrhea, being still another type of infection, can cause a discharge—although it is quite possible for women to have gonorrhea without recognizing symptoms.

The most important fact, to my way of thinking, is this: Any sort of irritation can cause a discharge. The various kinds are so common that the physician's first thought is to ask himself which type is present. The "social diseases" cause the minority rather than the majority of discharges. Perfectly innocent sources outnumber those related to any possible misbehavior.

What I seek to convey is that even the elderly maiden aunt should have no reluctance about reporting this annoying situation to her doctor. He knows from long experience that *anybody* can pick up one of these infestations, and the sooner they are treated, the sooner they cease to annoy.

The treatment often involves the use of a douche, frequently a mildly acid one (two tablespoons of vinegar to a quart of warm water). Special cases may call for more sophisticated medications, suppositories and powders. Currently, research scientists have been developing some medications that can be taken by mouth for some (but certainly not necessarily all) such cases. I don't have much hope that "a few pills" will ever be the answer to all these discharge problems, but I know that, even within my own lifetime, there have been tremendous additions to the treatments that are readily available and are highly effective.

How to Protect Yourself

In this chapter we have been talking as though a woman has special problems that a man does not have. That's right! But the opposite is true, too. Men are more subject to prostate troubles, to hernias (or ruptures), to heart disease earlier than are women, to a great deal more lung cancer. The average life span of a man is shorter than for a woman.

But the woman has her own special problems with the reproductive organs, the breasts, the difficulties of menopause, so we will continue this chapter as we began, strictly for women.

As a fundamental, remember that the normal state for women is painless. If menstrual cramps or other discomforts occur, they are not normal. They may not be and probably are not dangerous, but they are not something to be expected, not something that should be borne as the price of being a woman. The irritating discharges, the excessive swelling just before menstruation, the headaches at that same time—report them to your doctor so he can correct them.

Excessive menstrual flow is another such problem. It can contribute to anemia, besides being a thorough nuisance. Tell your doctor. See what can be done.

Irregular flow is another symptom that deserves attention. So, especially, does "spotting," or repeated, although small and un-expected, flow.

The "D. and C.," or dilation and curettage, is something which many women may never require—but no men will! This means a dilation of the cervix so that, with proper instruments, the inside of the uterus can be pared or "scraped." This is a common procedure.

Performed under anesthesia, it incapacitates a patient for only a few days. It is, however, a most extremely useful technique. Its principal but not its only purpose is diagnostic. In troublesome and continuing cases, more than one D. and C. may be necessary, and I hope to dispel the feeling that "I don't need another D. and C., because I've already had one." Your doctor, in many cases, will require more than one X ray or, for a simpler instance, may still take your temperature even though you "had your temperature taken yesterday." Understand my point?

The same D. and C., however, may also be curative in some cases. Uncontrollable bleeding may, for example, be due to a thickening of the lining of the uterus, some spot of tissue which was not completely ejected by the menstrual process. Curettage also is pretty much a fixed necessity after a miscarriage.

It is vitally useful in localizing suspected early cancer—and cancer of the uterus is second only to breast cancer as a cause of death among women.

We have every reason to believe that cancer of the uterus should be one of the least deadly of cancers, as curable as skin cancer, which can be cured in upwards of 95 percent of all cases if it is recognized early.

It is only among the uninformed that we find people who permit a skin cancer to go on and on before finally getting medical help, or who resort to quack cures in the belief that they can "burn the cancer out."

In the case of cancer of the uterus (or, more frequently, cancer of the cervix, or opening into the uterus) we have not had the advantage of being able to see the diseased spot developing.

Today, however, we have something even better than being able to see the cancer in its early stages. We can detect it even before it becomes large enough to see.

The method is the "Pap smear," named for its discoverer, Dr. George Papanicolaou, who died not so very long ago after seeing his discovery save literally thousands of lives.

A cancer, if it is where we can get at it, sheds abnormal cells that can be recognized under a microscope. A simple swabbing of the cervix provides a sample of the loose cells there. If some of them prove, under the microscope, to be cancerous, or even suspiciously on the border line, further examinations automatically follow. The "Pap test" is accurate in upwards of 90 percent of all cases. In the remainder, more precise tests are necessary.

This is where the D. and C. again becomes important. The discovery of abnormal cells, after a smear has been taken from the cervix, indicates that a cancer may be starting—somewhere. The assumption is that it is in the cervix, so biopsies are taken there—a biopsy being a needle-small sample of tissue.

If this is negative, as occasionally it will be, it may mean that the cancer is farther up, somewhere in the uterus. Here, as you can readily realize, the D. and C. becomes important. Little scrapings from any area that does not appear to be quite normal will provide ample numbers of cells for microscopic examination in the pathology laboratories.

Detected at this early stage, such cancers can be removed before they have a chance to spread. That is why, with the technical facilities we now have, cancer of the uterus, instead of being second deadliest, should almost disappear as a cause of death. In the last decade, the death rate has declined by about 30 percent. In the next decade, if we make use of what we know, we can reduce it by 90-odd percent instead of 30.

What is the message to women who read this? Have the simple, painless and not-very-expensive "Pap smear" as a routine safeguard. It should be done once a year after age 40, and some authorities prefer it every 6 months, which is that much safer.

Because this type of cancer has been observed to occur in some women 10 years earlier, plenty of conservative gynecologists and obstetricians think it should be started at age 30. I agree. If we are going to err, let's err on the safe side. But if one in a thousand such early tests detects a cancer early so that it can be completely eradicated to save a life, the odds are pretty good, I think. One chance in a thousand of saving a life! Or even if it is one in 10,000. But the odds aren't that long. The test will save more than that.

Just a few closing words on pelvic examinations, plus my own notions on pre-marital examinations, and in this I know that I am supported by a considerable number of my fellow physicians.

These last few paragraphs are needless to women who customarily have routine gynecological examinations and know that they are painless, that most physicians know that gentleness is in order and that with ordinary draping, exposure is minimal. The presence in the examining room of a nurse is reassuring—and this is usual practice.

Fear, nerves and tension not only make the procedure more difficult but can make it a bit painful. Relaxing and remembering that you are experiencing only what is routine for millions of others will make it a quick and occasional safeguard for your health.

As to premarital examinations, these usually are not much else but a blood test to determine whether syphilis is present. I'm all for detecting that—but ideally I think more than that ought to be included.

Why not a chest X ray for early signs of tuberculosis (and of some heart disease cases as an extra benefit)? Why not a urinalysis, which is rapid and inexpensive, to detect early diabetes plus, occasionally, the early case of kidney disease?

Whether a pelvic examination should be optional, I do not attempt to say, but as a father I think it would not be out of line and would avoid some future troubles early instead of allowing them to develop into critical troubles later.

I'm certainly no advocate of forcing everybody into a rigid pattern, but I do think that the general availability and acceptance of these tests would avert a great many of the subsequent heartaches that are recounted in the letters I receive.

14

WHAT YOU
SHOULD KNOW ABOUT SEX

MAXIM 14 *Sex is a normal part of life. Don't let false ideas ruin things for you.*

Sex is a perfectly natural part of our lives. Or at least it ought to be.

The fact seems to be that misconceptions, misapprehensions, old wives' tales, have become a terribly important factor in making life miserable for a good many of us.

I'm not at all sure but that true sex education for adults isn't, actually, a matter of unlearning things that aren't so, for a good many people.

If that sounds anomalous, think a minute. Animals, depending or instinct, seem to get along very well. Aboriginal tribes, not hampered by false modesty or childhoods warped by taboos, take sex in stride by "doing what comes naturally."

But in our complex civilization, further tangled by generations of making our children "learn about sex" from the forbidden whisperings of their almost equally troubled peers, we have managed to turn sex into a monster that causes an immense amount of needless harm—social and emotional harm, and sometimes some other kinds. Certainly health can suffer, if perhaps mostly as a secondary consequence of emotional upsets.

The twisted attitudes of youth sometimes are straightened out later. Sometimes the scars remain for life.

I am thoroughly aware of the concern, these days, over the apparent weakening of social codes, as regards sex, among our young people. Most certainly I am appalled at some of the recent statistics on venereal disease. I am willing to concede, for the sake of argument if nothing else, that our modern educational patterns, keeping young people in school longer than used to be the case, are a problem although I very much doubt—and we'll discuss this a bit later—that the difficulties are nearly as great as some people say, and I don't think they are at all insoluble.

None of these things seem to me, as a doctor, to lie at the root of this age's "sex problem."

No, the real "sex problem" seems to me to rest principally on these elements:

1. A refusal to think and talk about sex problems as matter-of-factly as we discuss diet, pure drinking water or any other universal aspect of living. No, we are still embarrassed, and whether knowingly or not, we continue to pass this hush-hush attitude on to our children, beginning in early childhood when we first begin evading the simple, sensible questions that little ones ask.

2. As a result, we leave our teen-agers pretty much adrift, picking up information and misinformation as best they can, but thoroughly aware that the hardest place to get any answers is at home.

3. Comes marriage, and while the majority find their way, gropingly, into a sensible sex relationship, some never do. Soaked in the sugary fiction of love stories, too many miss the real meaning of healthy sex and get it all mixed up with "romance," glamour and the stupid tape-measure notions of beauty which, in show business and beauty contests, have reduced beauty and sex attraction to statistics of circumference.

4. And finally a tremendously large sex problem has developed, little seen or heard, in our fully adult population.

This aspect, I must confess, had to a large degree escaped me, too, until I began writing a daily health column for newspapers a decade ago.

Every physician, of course, has more opportunity to see the signs of sex misunderstanding than does the average person. But even doctors, I realize now, can at best detect only a little of it. Embarrassment, lack of suitable words to express the problem, reluctance to ask for help with what seems to be such a personal problem—all these and other reasons seal the lips of people who would like to get some answers but can't bring themselves to ask.

But the newspaper column has been bringing home to me the amount of doubt, pain and anxiety that exists. These letters often begin:

> Dear Doctor Molner:
>
> I have a wonderful family doctor that we've been going to for years, but I just can't bring myself to ask him about this. . . .

WHAT PEOPLE ASK ABOUT SEX

I've had letters from readers aged from 13 to the seventies. Surprising as it may seem, the most frequent question involves frequency—or infrequency—of sexual intercourse.

> Dear Doctor:
>
> My husband is 70 and I am 68, and don't you think that at our age, five times a week is too often?

But for every letter like that, there will be half a dozen complaining of just the opposite.

> My husband is only 39 years old, but he might as well be 139 for all the good he is to me. He seems healthy, but don't you think there has to be something wrong with a man never to show any interest for months at a time? I have absolutely no reason to think he is interested in anyone else, but he just isn't interested in me.

From readers around 20 I get puzzled letters indicating how little, really, some of them know—in spite of our easy assumption that "the young people usually know more than we do, so why try to tell 'em?"

What about this really rather tragic plea:

> I am at present keeping steady company and plan to be married in the near future, and am quite at a loss to know just what is what—now and later. I will be anxiously watching your column. Please answer soon. George insists that since we are going to be married soon, I go all the way. Just what is "all the way"?

All right, friends, how do you answer a question like that? And how can you possibly cram into a newspaper column enough information to do that girl any good?

But that is a real letter, a real and despairing appeal for a stranger, writing a column in a paper, to explain the facts of life. Do our young people know more than we do? No, I think it's time we realized that some of them don't, and that it's up to us to help them. How? I'll get to that.

Still another question that comes to me, from time to time, is from a wife who has been urged into some act or other that her "moral" but vague upbringing has led her to believe is "wrong."

She agreed to it—but now she is overcome with remorse. She feels that she has done something "immoral" and is afraid that her husband will demand the same thing again. It has gotten so she resorts to all sorts of subterfuges to avoid any approach to love-making. In short, here's a marriage that may soon go on the rocks. Whether it winds up in the divorce court is not necessarily the question. The closeness, the frankness and friendship that marriage should imply, is gone. And both of them, their children and perhaps relatives and friends, suffer from this mysterious friction that has invaded the marriage.

From boys and young men, and perhaps even more often from older men, come questions about their virility. From a man in his fifties came this curious note, "Is a penis 5 inches long and an inch and a quarter wide in erection normal? Or is that an infantile type?"

I can imagine this man (can't you?) worrying about his "problem" from the time he was a teen-ager, and finally working up enough courage to ask his question decades later.

The answer to him, of course, is that he is normal enough. There are variations in all of us, from size of nose to size of feet. We don't worry about being able to walk because our feet happen to be size 5 or size 13. A small man may weigh 125 pounds. Another man may weigh three times that (although, of course, he's overweight!) But each earns a living, each recognizes that sheer size isn't the controlling element in life.

But because of the shroud of secrecy that surrounds much of the matters of sex, too many of us tend to worry or imagine that some fancied difference in us may be of tremendous significance. We dream up these bugaboos and let the worry fester, when in truth all we have to do is relax and admit that we're all just people, and we, like any other creatures, will do pretty well if we just do what comes naturally.

This, I truly believe, is perhaps the greatest "secret" there is in adjusting to a normal sex life—and it isn't a real secret at all. Yet in recent years I have become aware, as never before, of how many people are making themselves miserable by imagining all sorts of things that really don't matter.

The Real Meaning of Sex

Keep in mind that I am speaking as a physician, not a moralist, but when you get down to things of basic importance, you often discover to your own surprise that our forefathers weren't without sound reasons for establishing the moral codes that have survived the centuries.

It is unfortunate that "glamour" and sex have become such highly commercialized items in our society. Oh, I'm not a prude. I have no objection to "pin-up pictures." I don't go along with the self-appointed guardians of morality who object to a book because it may deal with sex, or, for that matter, even with immoralities. Literature isn't limited to the good in life. It is a reflection of life the way it is.

Neither am I astonished to discover that boys and girls do some kissing—and even some other things, which sometimes they shouldn't be doing. People were people when I was young!

But for all that, I also believe, on the basis of no inconsiderable evidence, that knowing of such things and accepting them as right are hardly the same thing.

Overemphasized sex too often is used to "sell" motion pictures, plays or novels to the public, yet a good deal of this "sales appeal" would vanish if we hadn't, some way or other, managed to endow sex with a label of being "forbidden."

No, sexual love is not a bad thing. It is a lovely thing and a necessary thing. It is the drive within us that perpetuates the human race. But it is a far cry from the real meaning of love to the hokum that fills some cheap fiction these days. It seems a pity that so many of our easy-reading mystery stories, the who-dunits, have been twisted into excuses to relate the affairs of characters who behave like tom cats that have been too long locked up. There is nothing real or believable about some of these potboilers, and they serve only to confuse our young people who don't realize how far from the truth they are.

True and enduring sexual happiness depends on love, on the desire of two people to share their lives, raise families, and learn to be as close together as two people can be.

Most certainly sexual love is not, as a few misled people seem to believe, only a means of perpetuating the race. It is, as well, an emotional, spiritual fulfillment. It is a part of life, just as beauty is a part of civilized life. To be sure, we could live in a tent or a shed, and survive without pictures or flower gardens or music. As far back as the days of the cave men, there was a groping urge to create art work, however rude and crude it was.

People aren't cattle. People aren't intended, like dogs or cats, to mate indiscriminately at such times as the female comes in heat. If for no other reason (although there are others, beyond the scope of this discussion), a home is a fundamental need for the human race. It may be a humble home. It may even be a home on wheels that moves constantly. But whatever it is, it is a home. Babies, unlike kittens, do not begin to fend for themselves at the age of a few weeks.

I'll leave it to the philosophers, the sociologists and the anthropologists to delve deeper into all of this. I'm interested only in pointing out that it is so.

Believe me, this becomes a matter of importance to a physician as he seeks to help patients who, strange as it may seem, haven't realized the deep significance of these facts. Many a time, by bringing out these points to people who thought they had a "sex problem," the difficulty has suddenly begun to iron itself out.

Satisfactory sex adjustment depends on the mutual love of two mature people. Mutual love and understanding overcome the obstacles that seem to be present when couples do not realize this but mistakenly think that sex is a matter of technique.

WHAT ABOUT THOSE WHO ERR?

Most of us, perhaps without realizing it, are brought up with the feeling that young people are better off if they wait to be married before engaging in sexual intercourse.

This I, too, believe. I have no ready answer for those who point out that young people, when they reach the age at which in some other societies they would already have been married, are under considerable pressure. This is true. For reasons of economics, extended education, military service and so on, our young folks are not always able to marry as soon as they reach physical maturity.

Yet promiscuity certainly is not the answer. There is too much of this, obviously. The rising tide of venereal disease is one sign. The number of children born out of wedlock is another.

But let me point out something that seems to have escaped many of the people who are seriously worried about these problems. The great mass of such cases is *not* among young people of 20 or a few years beyond. They, and I take this to be a good sign, have learned to take a sounder view. Some goodly numbers of them doubtless are engaged, looking forward to marriage and willing to wait.

No, the statistics show us that disease and illegitimacy are most dangerously high at ages several years lower, the sixteens and seventeens. There are varied reasons for this, I suspect, but we

cannot count among them the idea that there is any great deprivation in youngsters of this age getting along without the full
privileges of marriage.

Rather, too many of them are giving way, without any attempt
at restraint, to their desires. It may very well be that a good many
girls of that age, without any fully developed sexual urge as yet,
trade themselves for the ephemeral hope of being popular with
boys. It hardly needs saying that they do not achieve this, certainly not in any lasting way. Their reputations are soon tattered,
and the boys they might really want to marry aren't interested
in them.

I believe there is, as I hinted earlier, at least some element of
false values stirred up by the publicity that is attached to large-
busted entertainers—most of whom seem to have considerable
difficulty in maintaining their own marriages. There's a temptation to confuse the show-world emphasis on sex with real values.

I see no answer to these problems except education and a
general return, starting with early childhood, to acceptance of
moral precepts. And remember, please, that I am still talking as
a physician, not as a preacher. My concern is with the physical
and social wreckage, but some early-taught morality is at least
as important in the cure, I suspect, as some later-taught facts
about the dangers of promiscuity.

There is still another group for which at times I am even sorrier.
They are usually girls in the late teens or early twenties who have
gotten into sexual relationships, quite aware that they were not
condoned by society, but impelled by the various pressures that
sometimes develop.

True, many of these girls have escaped both disease and pregnancy, but too many times have I found them weighted down by
a sense of guilt. Sometimes it wrecks their schoolwork. Sometimes
it builds up such a burden that the emotional turmoil is reflected
in impairment of general health. The best I can tell them is to
return to heeding their consciences, but to put the past behind
them. The sense of guilt can perhaps last for years, upset lives
and damage marriages unless they can bring themselves to realize
that what is done is done, but that the future depends on how
they conduct themselves hence.

In this matter of guilt, there is one more thing that I certainly must mention, and that is masturbation. Here again we have a taboo subject, and the tacit agreement not to talk about it is leaving thousands of people in ignorance and, as a result, in fear and misery.

Some experts insist that all young men have masturbated. This is not far from the truth, in my estimation. If there are exceptions, they are few. Boys and young men write to me such pleas as "How can I save myself from this terrible thing?" Somewhere they have absorbed the idea that this is bound to ruin them morally, physically and mentally.

This simply is not so. Excessive indulgence can create a guilt complex of frightening proportions at times. But it has no effect on physical health. It does not stunt growth. It does not cause insanity. Carried to extremes, it may warp the attitudes toward sex life later on, and for this reason if for no other, a reasonable amount of self-restraint is wise. But like awkwardness, acne and daydreaming, this is a nuisance that young people seemed fated to have to get through, the best way they can, on the road to growing up.

Many a letter comes from an upset parent, in almost all cases a worried mother, who wants to know what she should do because she has discovered that her son has "acquired this evil habit."

There isn't anything to do, except ignore it. No good can come of storming, chiding, advising, shaming or anything else, and there can be harm—emotional—from fostering in the young fellow the idea that he is "wicked," is doing something that others haven't done. Just let the matter take care of itself, for it will.

The situation may be helped by diverting the boy's (or girl's) interests. Check on the books and magazines he may be reading; the type of movies he may be seeing. Try to get him physically occupied—a part-time job, more outdoor exercise, sports. This will take his mind off idle self-concern, and physical fatigue will promote more sound rest.

In the same category is worry over soiled bedclothes, the consequence of nocturnal emissions or "wet dreams." Here there is even less occasion to raise a storm. This is simply a sign that the young man is maturing. Unlike masturbation, it is an involuntary rather than a voluntary release of physical and emotional pressures that have been building within him. It is, by the way, possible for the emission to occur without any of the erotic dreams that often accompany them.

Perhaps still more alarmed are parents of babies or very young children who sometimes accidentally discover a pleasurable sensation in playing with their genitals. I can only counsel great caution and gentleness in dealing with this. Ignore it if this seems possible. At all events do not scold or punish. In some instances it may be found that this is more a reaction to chafing or tight clothing; more comfortable clothing may end the problem.

Girls, too, sometimes masturbate, not nearly as often as boys, to be sure, but sometimes. A letter that touched me very deeply was from a woman who described herself as "an old maid" in her fifties. In early childhood, before she had any idea of what it was all about, she admitted in the letter, she had begun masturbating and continued it for quite some years.

She should, of course, have realized that it was something that anyone might have encountered. But she didn't. She somehow got it into her head that she had transgressed some great moral law.

This, it seems, was the greatest reason why she never married. She even shut herself off from society to a large extent. So here she was, holding a job in a small town but having almost nothing to do with anybody, lonely, ashamed and frightened, when years ago if only someone could have impressed the truth upon her, she could have brushed it all into the past and gone about living a normal life.

A particular reason for her letter was that she had detected signs that some of her pelvic and urinary organs had shifted somewhat in position. This is not uncommon. Neither is it a difficult problem to correct. But this poor woman had it firmly fixed in her mind that this was a result of "self-abuse" when she was young, and that she would have to confess it all if she went to a doctor for care. Should she try to get a job in some other town, she asked, so she could get medical care where nobody would know her?

In the first place, masturbation, no matter what she believes, had nothing to do with her current troubles. Second, there is no occasion for her to bring that matter up when she talks to the doctor. Third, even if there *were* any bearing on the matter, and there isn't, it wouldn't matter to the doctor. Our purpose in life isn't to preach to people, or to judge them, but to help them.

The big tragedy, however, is that this woman's assumption of false guilt has made a mess of her life and destroyed her happiness for 30 or 40 years. And all because she didn't know; all because little scraps of misinformation are acquired by youngsters, and there is no opportunity to set them right.

LETTERS FROM MARRIED FOLK

By far the most frequent question in this matter from people of middle age is about the waning of sexual powers—or the reverse.

From Mrs. K. in Indiana:

> What's wrong with me? Too embarrassed to ask my doctor—why can't I enjoy my husband's love-making? I have always faked an interest, but inside I feel frustrated and tense. I feel sex in marriage is a sacred thing, a way of expressing love, not strictly passion. I am 52.

She's half right and half wrong, I should say. Yes, it *is* a way of expressing love, but it is a passionate expression of it.

I can only guess what lies behind any particular case, but a good many times it appears that the wife (sometimes the husband, but not often) is blocked by not being able to let go and relax and just enjoy love-making. It is very true that *love* is the important word, but I suspect that when the word *sacred* creeps in, it may mean that someone is missing the true realization that there must also be a naturalness.

Here's another:

> I am 19 and my husband is 21. I find I am frightened of intercourse. My mother would preach about girls who got in trouble. My husband blames my mother for the way I am.

So perhaps we must keep that in mind. It is one thing to teach our children proper behavior. It is another to lay on so much stress that they can't find pleasure in something that is right and natural and should afford overwhelming mutual satisfaction.

But it can be something else. Like this:

> I married at 17. My husband's brutal attempts at sex relations prostrated me so that I turned to masturbation. This marriage lasted 4 years. I have since remarried. He is a wonderful man. I have stopped the practice of masturbation.

There, in a little different sense, love is the key. A young husband may not be as skilled as one might want, but if love is the dominant emotion in his heart, he is never going to be guilty of being brutal about it. He can't.

But now to move along a few more years.

> My husband and I are in our sixties. I am in the mood to push him over a cliff. I would not care if I never heard the word "sex" for the rest of my life. My husband's attitude is affecting me psychologically and turning me against the act.
>
> He has a teen-age mind and will not face the fact that he is old and has lost his sex appeal if he ever had any. Instead of advice on sex to the young, let's have some for older folk, too.
>
> He finds me very desirable and gets upset when I can't respond as often as he thinks I should. Am I so abnormal?

No, I suppose she isn't—although from her letter I have no idea of the frequency with which he finds her "so desirable." The remark about his sex appeal "if he ever had any" would lead me to think that perhaps she always has been standoffish, and at long last now thinks that age should put an end to something she didn't like much in the first place.

Could I be right? Honestly, I don't know. I may be quite wrong in her case, but I am sure that the answer would be right for many. A certain proportion of women, if not frigid, are at least reluctant and submit from a sense of duty—which is entirely the wrong motive.

There is scant doubt that almost without exception these cases of frigidity are wholly emotional. They can be women who as children were lectured too hard, or were given false values, or were children of mothers who didn't like their fathers. There are countless similar situations. Frigidity is in the mind rather than being a physical matter. But the result is the same.

HUSBANDS WHO LOSE THEIR DRIVE

However hard it may be for such women to accept the fact, there are others who feel quite the opposite way.

Mrs. R. writes succinctly, "My husband is 60, looks 50, is active in sports, gardening, and works with real zip, but sexually he is dead. What happened?"

For every letter from a woman who would like to "push her husband off a cliff," there is at least one like that above—a woman who wonders where her husband's ardor went.

There are plenty of letters like one from Mrs. C. in Missouri:

> My husband has a problem—he has the urge for inter-course but is unable to have an erection. He is 54.

In complaints of this sort, both the physical and emotional factors may be at work—one or the other, or both at once.

The emotional factor is by far the larger. A man can become chronically fatigued, either because of some physical ailment or from sheer work. In the forties, fifties, even the sixties the demands of job, endless week-end chores around the house, worries, wrestling with the monthly bills and so on can be exhausting. We don't have the resilience of youth but the demands on our time, energy and nerves are even greater.

There is nothing unusual—it may well be the rule rather than the exception—for a man, reaching a certain level of tiredness, to feel that he just doesn't have the energy to make love. Or he tries and fails. And right there something worse happens to him. He is shaken and embarrassed by his failure. He begins to wonder whether he is "too old." There probably is no worse thought that can enter his head. Once he is unsure of himself, he has suffered about as hard an emotional blow as can exist in this matter. The more he worries, the less sure he is, and the less sure he is, the less chance he has of succeeding.

There is no ready answer for this—although there *are* answers.
The best practical rule I know is for him to quit trying.

That's right! Quit trying! And I hope that the wife of every
such man will read this, too, and comprehend. When he stops
trying to force himself, he relaxes and stops worrying. Or at least
stops worring so urgently.

It is then that some evening will come along when they've had
a good time, perhaps out to dinner, perhaps just playing pinochle
or fooling around with some hobby, or just watching TV, assuming that TV is having one of its better nights. Vacations with
change of scenery and environment also have an invigorating
effect.

Relaxed and with no thought of making love (and hence relieved of the pressure of worry), that's when powerful affection
suddenly sweeps up unannounced. And the problem is ended.

There are various ways a wife can knock the whole thing into
failure. She can keep urging him. She can "tactfully" say, "Well,
not tonight. But we will *tomorrow* night." She can complain. She
can laugh at him. She can be self-righteously martyred about it.
All of these will keep the pressure on him, and all you have to do
to keep him temporarily impotent is to keep the pressure on, keep
him trying to force himself, keep him worrying, keep him thinking that he "just has to" make good next time.

As an example of what this nervous pressure can do, a friend
of mine of notable vigor and attractiveness once told me what
happened to him when he was 19. He wasn't, I must confess, as
strictly virtuous as he might have been, and I'm afraid he still
isn't. But by now he has squired some of the world's famous
beauties, and I present his case not as one of impeccable behavior
but of sexual capability.

Anyway, he had, way back then, found a damsel who was both
attractive and willing, and he was overwhelmed to find that he
was completely helpless. His disappointment and alarm was
multiplied because she was a young lady upon whom he had been
lavishing considerable thought. He was looking forward to his
"conquest" with the greatest anticipation.

Next day he went to a doctor. (I wish I knew who the wise old
fellow was, but that fact has been lost in the mists of memory.)

"Something terrible has happened to me . . ." the young fellow began, and he described his abject failure.

The old doctor grinned and said, "Young man, it's happened to everybody. You were all keyed up. That's what happens, that's what happens. Maybe you're lucky. You found out early what nerves can do."

And it's true. Just put in the back of your mind some worry—well, *worry* isn't exactly the word—or thought of interruption. A phone call is likely. Or maybe some night-owl friends might stop by. Or your head is full of worries and plans about what has to be done tomorrow. The youngsters are restless or may barge in. Just keep yourself worrying about something, or your mind cramped onto some problem or other, and you've given yourself a superb chance of failure.

There are a couple of other items, other than nerves and weariness. Substantial overweight is (or can be) a factor in impotence, and a doctor, when the problem has been brought to his attention, may logically put a man on a reducing diet. It may well be that the emotional aspect again plays its part. *Expecting* the reducing to help is part of the battle. But just getting down toward normal weight has a very real effect.

Faulty eating in general can do its damage, too. I am not by any means saying that just swallowing a vitamin pill is going to do any good, but if a man has gotten into the habit of subsisting on unbalanced meals, he's going to pay for it. He will pay for it more ways than this, of course. But then, I've made mention elsewhere that sensible eating pays health dividends.

Finally, and perhaps not the smallest item, there's alcohol. Alcohol is a depressant. An important one. Yes, it can relax you. Yes, it can release inhibitions. But beyond that, it can also deaden the senses and retard activity to the extent that you're not good for much of anything. Including love-making.

THE LADIES' SIDE OF THINGS

There have been plenty of discussions as to which is "the stronger sex." In this, as in some other aspects (just take longevity for one) the female seems to be the more rugged of the species.

Man, as I have so candidly exposed, can indeed be a delicate flower, rendered helpless simply because his tender nerves undermine his sense of esteem, his self-assurance.

From age 6 to 96, the male can be turned into an abject, tongue-tied, gauche critter by the calculated phrase of a woman.

Please do not ask me why. That's beyond my province, and I gladly leave it to be analyzed by those who think they can. But it seems to be true.

On the other hand, the female of the species, while more emotionally rugged and powerful, seems also to be vastly more sensitive. Sensitivity and strength are not opposites. They are not even antagonists. They are quite separate qualities.

Who but a man can come in from the backyard, feet muddy, whiskery, smelly, wearing his old clothes, and think that he is a supermasculine being calculated to make his wife swoon with delight that he notices her?

Sounds silly, doesn't it? It is. But I'm no exception. I've felt that way. So, I suspect, has almost every male. I do not expect our wives to understand our peculiar attitude. But after some consideration of the matter, I'm dratted if I can see any reason why our wives should sink meltingly into our arms under such circumstances.

Making love is important to women. It is a time for delicacy. It is a time for beauty and sweetness. Of coaxing and kissing and petting. And why we man-critters think that the messy and sweaty signs of our maleness make us irresistible, I don't know. After a good many years of thinking it over, the only reasonable conclusion I can achieve is that in this matter we are damn fools.

Physiologically, the female likes and needs to be nicely coaxed and cajoled along. She needs to be told that she is lovely and wanted. She doesn't want to be the aggressor. She wants to be so desirable that her man can't help being the aggressor. That's her nature. If he has any sense (and I suppose most of us mere men don't have any) he'll make her know that for him she is the prettiest, enticingest, most lovable woman who ever walked the earth.

To my fellow males, let me add this. I haven't by a whit departed from what I said earlier in this chapter. The base, the heart, the essence of sex is love. You married this wife of yours because for you she was, and still is, all these things. She is the one you want above all others, above all else in life. You can argue as much as you please that by this time she ought to know it. She ought to realize that if you didn't love her, you wouldn't have married her in the first place. Your logic no doubt is entirely valid. But it doesn't make any imprint on the mind of your beloved wife. She wants to be told. So tell her! I offer you no medical or scientific proof for this because I don't have any. But I submit that this makes at least as much sense, and probably a lot more, than the persistent male figment that whiskers, no socks and rumpled clothes make a man fascinating.

We men, I note, are quick enough to say that our wives aren't at their best in pin curls, wrinkled wrappers and run-over slippers.

And here's another problem which has come to me in enough letters to convince me that it is important. The act of love-making certainly is not just a simple, passion-impelled incident, as it is with some animals. The odor of perfume, the touch of a hand, the sound of music, the caress, the gentle "love bite,"—these are just a few samples of the things that translate into love language.

How you hold your beloved, what you may do and what you may not do, these, too, are part of it. I have had at least enough letters to disturb me from spouses (usually wives) who say that their husbands wished to do this or that. At least in the letters to me, wives have sometimes agreed but with misgivings and afterward complained that they "didn't think it was right." And the smoldering battle was on.

This is a rather delicate point for me to try to discuss here, within the limited space of a chapter. I suggest that people read any of the fairly numerous and sound books available on the subject of sex. There isn't very much that a sensible, reasonable couple would consider doing that is likely to be harmful. Sex is a matter of what you mutually wish to do together, and, with few exceptions, whatever you want to do is all right.

But I can't refrain from adding this, and emphatically: The word *mutual* is the important word. What may be enjoyable for one couple can be repugnant to another couple. Or repugnant to just one member of the marriage.

There is essentially nothing about sex that cannot be answered by resorting to the most important rule of all: Love. What does my beloved want? What does my beloved *not* want?

You can write a million words, or a million books, and you can ask limitless questions. But there are essentially none that will not be answered, and correctly answered, by applying the rule of love. How can I bring happiness to the one I love.

There is no better rule.

IF YOU CAN'T HAVE CHILDREN

At this point I want to spend a little time, at least, on the subject of sterility, real or imagined.

For all the words now being devoted to birth control, letters from my newspaper readers indicate a great deal more concern with just the opposite, the inability to have children. Perhaps it is because by now most people feel they already know whatever they want to know about birth control. But when, instead, the difficulty is in encouraging conception, they need and ask for help.

True sterility is a far less common thing than many suppose. That is to say, there are, indeed, cases in which one partner or the other is permanently unable to become a parent. Far more often, however, the "sterility" is something that may be corrected. Or, again, it is a relative matter. Fertility may not be up to par, but it is not entirely absent. Often it can be bolstered.

Finally there are cases in which we cannot ascribe any specific reason, yet we know, from long observation of such problems, that the emotions in some way play an important part.

For an example of this, one couple had tried for years to have a baby without success. All known tests indicated that there was nothing physically wrong. At last the couple decided to adopt a baby.

And what happened? Immediately after that they began having a series of three of their own! We can only assume that once the pressure was off, once they no longer were so intently trying to have a baby, Nature finally responded.

However, in the way of general rules for people who want babies, here are the suggestions, time-tested, that will bring the most success with the least waste of time, money and worry.

First: Since the days of Henry VIII and doubtless long before him, it has been popular to blame any lack of fertility on the wife.

Scientifically, there is nothing to this. It is simply a manifestation of the male ego, a hand-me-down from the times when the husband was the lord and master of everything, regardless of whether he made any sense.

The fact is that there's about as much chance one way as the other. The husbands are the sterile ones at least as often as the wives.

Since it is simpler, quicker and, hence, less expensive to test the husband first, that is the place to start. Many a virile male may object—but when you get right down to facts and logic, that's the place to start. Essentially, a sperm test is the heart of this examination. If they are sufficiently numerous, and healthy, and have motility—the ability to move around—they have all the characteristics they need. If they are deficient in any of these respects, then the search has to go farther, and find out why, and whether it can be corrected.

The initial examination, however, tells whether attention should be focused on the husband, or whether examination should shift to the wife.

If the latter, then a variety of elements need to be investigated: Whether the Fallopian tubes, through which the ovum or egg must move from the ovaries, are scarred, kinked or plugged; whether they can be reopened; whether there are fibroid tumors that can militate against conception; whether there is an excessively acid condition in the vagina; whether some condition of the uterus, such as endometritis, needs treatment.

When the essentials are known to be present, then the goal is to achieve the correct timing.

The ovum, as it leaves the ovary, is capable of being fertilized within a span of something like 48 hours. This may vary somewhat, but that is about the time.

It is, therefore, necessary that the sperm reach and fertilize the ovum sometime within that limited period. But how to know when that is? Roughly speaking, the ovum begins its descent through one of the Fallopian tubes approximately midway between the beginning of the last menstrual period and the beginning of the next.

Keep in mind, however, that this is not a rigid timetable that can be depended upon as you can depend on a commuter train. The average menstrual cycle is 28 days, but it can, without being abnormal, be considerably longer. It can vary, because of stresses of various sorts, in an individual from one month to another. While one ovum usually is produced each time, it is occasionally possible for more than one to be released.

For these and other reasons, pregnancy, at least theoretically, can occur at considerable different times, but that is another matter. What concerns us here is that the 48 hours, or less immediately after ovulation (the emergence of the ovum from a follicle in the ovary) is, decidedly, the time of maximum fertility.

For the woman who is extremely regular in her cycle, it is rather easy to anticipate this fertile time. For the woman whose cycle fluctuates, it is not so easy.

Here, however, another method becomes useful. That is keeping a record of daily temperature. (For this, rectal temperature will be preferable.) There will be, with ovulation, a slight increase in temperature of perhaps half a degree or more.

True, a cold, fatigue, the strain of staying up late for a gay party—such things can cause fluctuations in temperature, too, but after you have kept a chart of daily temperatures for a couple of months or so, you begin to have a pretty good idea of when ovulation is causing this increase.

That is the time at which the ovum is most likely to accept fertilization. Indeed, for the strongest chance of success, count it as the first 24 rather than the first 48 hours.

I have known of couples who followed this advice with perhaps too much literal-mindedness. There have been wives (and will be more, I am sure!) who have noted the sudden rise in temperature and even phoned their husbands to hurry home from work!

Yes, some are fortunate enough to be able to take time off whenever they wish.

There is, however, some added leeway. The spermatozoa also have a viable period. It probably is no more than perhaps two days in the genital tract, but the fact remains that impregnation a short time *before* ovulation offers a reasonable chance of success. Therefore, for practical purposes, and if you are blessed with reasonably regular cycles, anticipating the time of ovulation by perhaps a day can be effective.

A few women who suffer a brief but sometimes rather sharp pain at the time the follicle ruptures and the ovum begins its brief time of viability, can interpret that as a sign of the time at which fertility is maximum.

In addition to the aforementioned factors, it is more than worthwhile to remember that other less specific matters can have a distinct effect on fertility.

Underactive thyroid, a condition that can be readily treated medically, has been determined by many a doctor to be a factor in inhibiting conception. This can apply either to the wife or husband, possibly somewhat more to the husband.

Faulty nutrition, just not eating balanced meals which provide a full complement of vitamins and minerals, seems to be involved at times.

Most decidedly, chronic fatigue and nervous stress may be factors. Mankind wasn't intended to live in long, unrelieved periods of hard work, curtailed sleep and tension.

There are, of course, some more abstruse elements which may be involved, but I think you will find that the above is a reasonably concise outline of the principal considerations. If more complicated and difficult matters may enter in an occasional case, I can only say that you will have to rely on the observations and advice of a specialist anyway.

But when, or if, you are told, as must happen in some cases, that it is impossible or extremely unlikely that you can have children, I would accept the verdict, difficult as it may be. There is no use chasing will-o'-the-wisps. If you want children, then the recourse is to adopt. Don't put that off too long, because the agencies handling such matters quite rightly prefer to put little babies in the care of foster parents who are still fairly young.

I might add that an adopted child soon becomes so dear that the foster parents think of the child just exactly as they would one of their own. And the baby, growing up in an atmosphere of such love, may know that he is adopted but loves his adopted parents just as truly and deeply as he could possibly love his own.

15

STORM SIGNALS OF HEALTH

MAXIM 15 *Know the danger signs to look for; but also know how to stop worrying about things that don't matter. And by all means learn to recognize the quack methods and the old wives' tales.*

It would be handy, wouldn't it, if we could have two or three tests that would tell whether our health is good or whether something is out of balance and needs attention.

Handy—but hardly reasonable.

This very notion, however, is the basis for one of the hardy perennials of quackery. Knowing the respect which all of us naturally have for the scientific advances of recent decades, the charlatans have contrived various machines that are supposed to diagnose whatever condition may exist in the body.

It is perfectly true, of course, that we now use all sorts of sophisticated instruments to tell us things about the body and its state of health that we could discover in no other way. We can detect, observe and measure the faint electric currents in the brain—the EEG or electroencephalograph. We can do the same with the heart—the EKG (or ECG) or electrocardiograph. We can use X ray to "see" inside the body. With microscope or chemical tests we can get correct answers from tiny samples of materials pertinent to diagnosis. We are able to differentiate micro-organisms—germs, cells, fungi or protozoans.

We learn from sounds—the stethoscope. We can measure the blood pressure, count the pulse, take the temperature, determine (from a basal metabolism or other test) the rate at which we use up our food.

We can take a drop of blood, or a few drops of urine, or a sample of coughed-up sputum, or some moisture from a mucous surface, and derive very accurate conclusions from it. We can tap a patient's knee with a little rubber hammer and watch the reflex. We can send a trace of blood to the laboratory and in a day or two learn how rapidly it responds to an electrical stimulus. This provides us with definite diagnosis of some diseases which used to require (and I am not exaggerating) several weeks of observation and simpler tests before we could be sure what was happening.

All these are real, reliable, honest.

A good many of them sound like black magic unless we have studied the principles upon which they depend.

The fact that such scientific devices can be used for diagnosis is the very fact that has been diverted to the devious purposes of the quacks. They set up impressive-looking machines with electrical meters, meaningless lights, switches and other such gadgets and then assure trusting people that the apparatus can tell whatever the matter is, from asthma to neuritis. Some have used electrical contacts, some have claimed to make such broad-range diagnoses from a blood sample. One quack was unmasked when he gave a "diagnosis" with a sample actually taken from a dead chicken!

An informed person, of course, will not be taken in by these fanciful swindles. So—be an informed person.

There isn't any method, machine or technique that can make a complete examination of a person's health that way. Any time such a claim is made, beware. Better yet, report it to the police or to the Food and Drug Administration, which is perpetually hunting out quacks.

Some of the "sales pitches" used for these curious devices must be very convincing. At any rate, they keep on victimizing the public. If you happen to be tempted sometime to believe them, keep the modern airplane in mind.

You know that scores upon scores of gauges are required merely to keep track of the mechanical functioning of the plane in ordinary flight. In addition to this, the engines are torn down and rebuilt regularly after a fixed number of hours of operation.

That gives us some sort of idea of the checking required for a piece of machinery. Yet the human body is so vastly more complicated. Because of the power of living organisms to renew themselves, cell by cell, the body is also far more durable than an airplane. The human body, after all, continues for 50, 75 or 100 years.

But this does not mean that it is any less intricate. Quite the reverse! And thus it is that no single, all-inclusive means exists for "measuring" or assaying the total health of the body.

How Do We Judge Health, Then?

For everyday purposes, the best guide to our need for medical attention is the most obvious one: We feel ill. Or we "don't feel up to par." Or we don't see properly or hear properly. Or—a most useful safeguard for us—there is pain.

For somewhat long-range matters, we have some other valuable tip-offs: unaccountable loss of weight, undue fatigue and listlessness, a chronic cough, continuing fever, "night sweats," bleeding without apparent reason, lumps or growths, abnormal shortness of breath.

It is natural for us to recognize most of these signs—all of them, I hope, with perhaps two or three exceptions. Every so often a letter like this one arrives at my desk:

> Dear Doctor:
>
> What can I do about perspiring at night? I wake up wringing wet, even though the room is not too warm and I don't have too many covers on the bed.

This may be more than just an uncomfortable nuisance. These "night sweats" may be a warning of unrecognized infection somewhere in the body, a portent that serious trouble may be in the offing.

True, other causes may sometimes be at work, but it is a sign that should not be ignored. The question that comes readily to a physician's lips is this: "How long since you have had a chest X ray?" For many of us, knowing the advances that have been made in the war on tuberculosis, sometimes forget that there is still a great deal of it remaining, and that nobody is absolutely safe from it. No longer is the diagnosis of tuberculosis so close to being a sentence of death, as used to be the case. Quite the contrary. The great majority of TB victims now recover. But they don't get well without treatment, and the sooner they start it, the sooner they will be well and the fewer friends and relatives they will unknowingly make ill.

Nor is TB "a young person's disease." Each year it moves in the opposite direction—or we let it. The older person, especially the older man, steadily becomes a more important peril in spreading the disease. Grandpa's hacking cough may not be from his smoking or from bronchial trouble (a frequent but possibly erroneous supposition). So add the cough to the night sweats as an oft-neglected symptom.

Tuberculosis, besides remaining a very serious menace, is also a prime example of the type of disease which does not make the patient noticeably ill in the beginning. Nor is it confined entirely to the lungs. The tuberculosis organism is a germ; it can perpetrate different kinds of mischief, depending on where it attacks. It can attack the bones, the brain and other areas. In passing, it is worth comment that when I first entered medicine, tuberculosis meningitis was 100 percent fatal. Today most such patients are saved by use of anti-TB drugs.

Anyway, the increasing question today is how best we can detect the diseases which come on gradually. We have pretty well learned the lesson of how to combat and largely prevent the wholesale killers of other years: smallpox, typhoid, diphtheria, a good deal of the pneumonia. No wonder we are now having to pay more attention to the slowly developing problems, such as cancer, heart disease, atherosclerosis, high blood pressure, kidney and liver diseases, strokes.

THE WAY TO FIND THE SIGNS

We'll discuss, in a moment, a little about how to find the early signs of the diseases which don't make themselves suddenly and unmistakably known. Before doing so, let's see if there isn't something to be learned from the conquest of the older scourges.

How did we conquer typhoid, diphtheria and smallpox? Not by finding cures for them, but by preventing them. All of these diseases remain dangerous. All of them, while subdued, recur occasionally in the United States.

Why and how do they occur? Only through our neglect. Smallpox, when occasionally we hear of a case, is the result of someone not keeping his vaccination effective. The same is true for diphtheria. Typhoid breaks out (as we noted in that disastrous episode in Switzerland) when a community does not follow through with the knowledge we already possess about keeping water (or milk) supplies pure.

It becomes somewhat shocking to a physician to hear someone (and this *does* still happen) say, "I don't need a vaccination. The scar from the one I had in school in still perfectly plain."

The scar is of no significance. The question is: What about the antibody level in the blood, the ability of the blood to destroy the particular germ in question? We have, and have had for some time, the makings of some dangerous epidemics if certain of these diseases ever get a good start. Adults, required to have a smallpox vaccination, often are surprised to find that they have a "take."

A "take" means that they had lost their immunity to smallpox. This happens often enough to make it clear to any doctor that there must be a great many people whose immunity has worn off. I hope we never have enough smallpox cases filtering into our country to get a good start among such people, because the disease could pass from one unsafe individual to another until the total result would be devastating.

So before we go on to the signs to watch for regarding our health, let's first of all be sure that we are making use of the safeguards which already exist, our inoculations against smallpox, diphtheria, polio, tetanus. They don't last forever, but it is easy and inexpensive to have boosters every several years.

Once we have seen to that, it is time to think about the less explosive elements.

It is pretty generally known by now that many large corporations require that their executives have searching health examinations every year or so. (This may mean one or more days of the executive's time while he is being X-rayed, blood-tested and examined.) We know by now that such procedures do indeed turn up clues to conditions which are beginning to develop. We also are aware that a great deal of the testing doesn't show anything wrong. It just shows normality. And we also know that the cost may be beyond the means of most of us.

Do we need testing programs of this sort to be healthy? No, I don't think so. These multiple, specialized batteries of tests are a luxury, or perhaps we should say that they are an expensive sort of insurance to protect the companies from the unexpected loss of highly trained executives.

It is not absolute insurance. There is no method, no matter how complicated or how costly, which can anticipate all of the health problems which *might* arise. But for a very modest investment we can find most of them. This process of exhaustive examination is a matter of diminishing returns. If we make the basic tests, we detect most of the troubles quite readily. Beyond that, we get into the luxury classification, adding the tests which might, once in a while, give us slightly earlier detection of some few ailments.

WHAT YOUR DOCTOR SEES

The average patient would be flabbergasted if he had any idea how much his doctor sees in a matter of minutes. Many of the things are anything but abstruse. How is the patient's color? How does he sit or stand or walk? Is he brisk or tired? Posture good? Weight? Alertness?

The doctor takes your pulse—and in the process notes any unusual dryness or moistness of your skin. He takes a look at your fingernails. Any streaks or ridging? He may pinch a finger—and watch to see how quickly the color returns afterward.

With a stethoscope he learns about your heart—and also about the sounds of your breathing. Another minute or two and he has your blood pressure. He may or may not feel that a cardiogram is necessary. A look into your eyes (as we've discussed in an earlier chapter) can tell a lot of things that have no relation to your eyesight.

A blood test, allowing time for the laboratory work to be done, adds more data. A urinalysis gives a clue not only to that frequent ailment, diabetes, but to signs of kidney or bladder disorders. If anything looks suspicious, a further and more definitive test is in order.

We could go on, but that's a fair beginning. Add to this such things as you have noted: any difficulty in swallowing, digestive disturbances or any of the basic symptoms we listed earlier.

Certainly you won't fall into the habits of the sort of patient who presents himself at the office with the attitude of "Here I am. Now you tell me what's wrong." This isn't a guessing game. And it isn't for the doctor's benefit. If you've noticed something, tell your doctor. Don't waste everybody's time, including your own, by rattling off the details of your stubbed toe. But if your foot still hurts afterward, have the doctor take a look. If you break out in a rash every time you eat strawberries, then quit the strawberries. But if you think there's a lump developing, tell your doctor.

If you are pretty tired after having stayed up until 3 A.M., that's not news. But if you have dizzy spells or brief blackouts when you stand up suddenly, it's worth mentioning. It may not mean anything dangerously wrong, but it may tie in with some other item of fact in the examination.

Don't overestimate or underestimate the effect of your emotions. Fatigue, in itself, is natural, a signal that you need more rest, or perhaps need a vacation. It may also be a signal that you are not being very bright about your eating. Poor nutrition is a very common cause, especially in women. Skimping on breakfast is no way to reduce. Neither is it a good way to save time for your household duties—because saving 10 or 15 minutes hardly recompenses you for a whole morning of dragging around, too tired to enjoy life. A breakfast containing adequate protein—eggs and/or bacon, sausage or ham, some milk and some toast—cures a lot of these cases. And I mean just what I say. It cures a lot of them.

If, despite sensible eating and getting enough sleep, you still are unduly tired all the time, it may mean that some tests of your thyroid are in order. But it also may mean that you are chewing your reserves of energy to pieces with emotional turmoil.

The psychological factors—boredom, apprehension, job frustration, anxiety, suppressed worries whether over your health, your home, your children or whatever—take their toll.

Insomnia? Experience has taught me to be pretty cautious about this complaint. This applies even to the patient who says that he (or she) "heard the clock strike every hour from 11 o'clock to 7 this morning." This may be so, but it doesn't mean that the patient didn't get a fair night's rest. By now this has been tested out a great many times in hospitals, and the patient who "didn't sleep a wink" has been found gently snoring at all the periodic observations taken by the nurses.

No, I do *not* mean that the patient is untruthful. Some, and perhaps quite a few, subconsciously rouse themselves periodically in the night, hear a clock or look at a watch, and are totally unaware that they have still been sleeping 50 minutes out of each hour.

Besides that, our need for sleep is not fixed. As we get older there is less physical exertion, and in many cases it may not be necessary to get seven or eight hours of sleep. Five or six, if it is restful sleep, may be enough. But it depends on the individual, on how strenuous his day is, on his natural needs, on the nervous tensions of his day.

HOW TO CHECK FOR CANCER

Heart, circulatory and malignant ailments, in that order, are the ones of highest mortality today. The fact that cancer rates third (not first, as many believe) may be somewhat aside from the main point. Heart and circulatory diseases, with a good many major exceptions, often develop far in advance of the time at which substantial treatment or prevention is attempted. The fellow who for the last 30 or 40 years has spent most of his time sitting down can't make up for it by resorting to exercise after he is too old and too fat, and his heart has suffered too much. Exercise, beyond a mild degree, will be more perilous than helpful in many cases.

Or let's put it this way. To take care of our hearts and arteries, we should begin early in life, acquiring the habits of eating and exercising and resting and keeping our tensions within reason. The longer we ignore these simplicities, the less we can do later on to combat the consequences.

Cancer, however, is different. For the most part we do not know how to avoid cancer—with the exception of not smoking, and a few specialized aspects of certain types of cancer. We cannot predict it. But unlike heart disease in some of its basic aspects, we can quite often cure it completely—assuming that we find it and treat it in time.

We now cure something like one case of cancer in three, and there is very good reason to think that with our present knowledge, if we use it all, we can cure every other cancer.

Using the knowledge we now possess starts with the patient himself. For one thing, he (or she) must make use of the tests now available. The "Pap test" for cancer of the cervix has saved a great many lives, but probably no test we have can promise a greater increase in lives that can be saved from now on. We have done no more than make a good start in its use.

We can save other lives by reporting the early patches of what seem to be thickened skin, or other such painless abnormalities in the mouth. We can save still others by *never* letting a curious "sore that doesn't hurt" exist on the skin without being examined. Still other lives can be saved by investigating lumps in the breast immediately. Most of them will not be cancer; some of them will. The only way to be sure is to examine them all. And there are still other cancers, of lesser frequency, which can be arrested successfully if detected in time.

Rectal examination, preferably with a proctoscope, is an important safety precaution. The patient should also report any sign of bleeding, or any marked and continued change in bowel habits, but the proctoscope examination usually will give an earlier warning. Hoarseness or change in the voice or irritation or cough can mean cancer of the larynx. The same symptoms may mean something else, but unless you look, you can't know.

Stomach cancer may be suspected when there is loss of appetite, loss of weight, or chronic stomach distress. X-ray examination is essential. Other signs of cancer there or elsewhere may be unexplained fever, anemia, abnormal sedimentation rate (another type of blood test), certain enzyme studies. Enlarged lymph glands warn of some other cancers.

It is quite obvious that every symptom I have mentioned can be the result of something other than cancer. But I hope you will keep this thought in mind, too. Every symptom I have mentioned is the result of *something*.

If we paid adequate attention to every one of the routine warning signs for cancer, we not only would cure a great deal more cancer, but we would be able to cure a considerably larger number of other diseases.

AN UPSIDE-DOWN CHECKLIST

So with that in mind, let me list the famous "seven danger signals," and with them a few of the noncancerous causes of them.

I do this with the mental reservation that perhaps some readers will attach themselves to the possible nonmalignant causes and thus excuse themselves—in deadly fashion—from having the signs investigated. Yet such excessively cancer-fearing individuals will be ostriches anyway, sticking their heads in the sand rather than looking at the facts.

There may, I trust, be a considerably larger number of readers who will say to themselves, "Well, I guess maybe Dr. Molner may have a point or two on his side," and find this a good reason for checking on symptoms at once instead of dreading and delaying.

Most of us do, I think, have a habit of going to extremes. We either expect the worst, or we go the other way and tell ourselves that "It's nothing at all. It will clear up by itself."

The truth, in a very large proportion of cases, will lie somewhere between, and the trouble will be something that can be corrected readily. So here are the "seven danger signals" with reverse emphasis:

1. "Any sore that does not heal." But this can also be an ulcer, an infection of some sort, some form of dermatitis, a place being irritated by a jagged tooth.

2. "A lump or thickening in the breast or elsewhere." As a matter of plain statistics, enlarged glands are benign and far outnumber malignant growths. It is my belief that most lumps in the breast should be removed for microscopic study, because the occasional malignancy that will be found outweighs the effort involved. And anyway, removal of a lump, even though benign, is of benefit. It does not mean removing or mutilating the breast, either. Lumps elsewhere can be cysts (which are numerous, temporarily swollen glands), enlarged tendon sheaths, lipomas (harmless "fatty tumors"), and a host of other things.

3. "Unusual bleeding or discharge." Intestinal or rectal bleeding may be from an ulcer, diverticulitis, hemorrhoids, fissures. All of these need treatment and are not likely to "get better by themselves." Discharges of other kinds more likely will indicate infection—again a condition which needs treatment, and the sooner it starts the easier it will be.

4. "Any change in a wart or mole." This means any change in size, shape or color. It means any tendency to bleed or have a raw appearance. Many times it will actually amount only to some irritation—a strap, buckle, belt or collar chafing it. Removal of these small surface blemishes is simple. It also eliminates the risk of continued irritation ultimately leading to a real cancer. But when these blemishes are not irritated and show no sign of change, they may be safely left alone.

5. "Persistent indigestion or difficulty in swallowing." Naturally persistent indigestion doesn't necessarily mean cancer—but who wants persistent indigestion? (See chapter on the digestion for ramifications of this.) Nor does difficulty in swallowing necessarily stem from any single cause. Pressure, as caused by enlarged glands in the neck, or sheer nerves (as many a high-strung person has discovered) or pressure from a benign tumor are among the many causes of difficulty in swallowing. Again, correction is re-

quired—or if it is just a matter of nerves, finding that out can be all that is needed to let the patient's nerves relax a bit.

6. "Persistent hoarseness or cough." Smoking, a sore throat, emphysema, asthma, allergies and lung disorders such as tuberculosis or fungus infection are a few of the possibilities. Cancer of the larynx or lung can mimic them all.

7. "Any change in normal bowel habits." Colitis, food allergies, incorrect changes in eating habits, adhesions—and you could go on and on. Irregularity in bowel habits is neither good for you nor comfortable.

In short, the seven danger signals for cancer are likewise danger signals for many, many other conditions, and if you keep the signs in mind, you will have gone a long way toward guarding your health generally.

MAKE UP YOUR MIND SLOWLY

It is the exception rather than the rule, anyway, that a patient is either wise or correct when he goes to a doctor with his mind all made up as to what is causing his trouble. For one, the patient cannot help but be subjectively swayed. He can't be dispassionate about weighing the symptoms. For another, there is the perfectly human impulse to note the presence of one or more symptoms and jump to the conclusion that they indicate a certain disease process.

Diagnosis isn't that simple. Having *some* of the symptoms fit the disease isn't enough. They all have to fit. If some don't fit, then another diagnosis is indicated. It is the doctor's task to keep that always in mind. It has been a cardinal rule of his training from the beginning.

Lest I seem to be saying that patients don't have sense enough to know what is going on—that is *not* what I mean, because doctors themselves often have experienced the same thing. We've all been sure we had every disease in the book as we went through medical school. I dare say it was good for us. It taught us, the hard way, that a few symptoms don't tell the story.

Some of us have fallen into the same error, in moments of panic, later on. I plead guilty to it myself. Once I was thoroughly certain that I had serious heart trouble and told one of my colleagues. "Show me exactly where the pain is," he told me. I did so.

"That takes care of that," he said, and grinned. "When you can point to the exact spot, then it isn't your heart, is it?"

The person who treats himself has a fool for a doctor, so the saying goes, and it is true whether the patient be layman or doctor.

Chest pain is quite a common occurrence, and I suppose we all must have a natural tendency to wonder whether it isn't the heart. Again, there are numerous other causes: muscle strain, intercostal neuralgia, "referred pain" from a pinched nerve, hiatal hernia, shingles. Appetite depressant drugs can cause chest pain. So can excessive smoking. Chest injuries involving the cartilage attachments of ribs and breast bone can be painful for a long time.

Nor is our old friend, nervous tension, to be lightly dismissed. I have in mind a former athlete (later a successful business man) who had persistent chest pains for weeks. He fell into the error of shopping from one doctor to another. Each one, on the basis of initial examination, had different notions as to what the trouble *might* be, but this peregrinating patient never went back often enough to the same doctor to permit finding out for sure. Besides, his symptoms had a way of changing. His chest always hurt, but never exactly in the same place or the same way.

One of his friends finally built up a story about a particular surgeon being a great authority on the chest. He also tipped off the surgeon about the background of the whole worrisome affair.

Thus forewarned, the surgeon nodded very gravely, asked a lot of questions which were designed not to give the patient any hints (some of the questions made sense and some of them, frankly, were window dressing for this particular case), and finally administered some mild sedatives.

The chest pains began to ease almost at once. It wasn't until afterward that the patient learned what really ailed him. He was so tense and jittery that he succeeded in giving himself some muscular cramps!

Just as I have warned earlier not to leap to the conclusion that you have some dreaded disease, equally I must warn that tension isn't to be attributed as the cause until the evidence supports such a conclusion.

The long and short of it remains this:

Tell your doctor your symptoms—and by now you have a general idea of the principles. Then leave the diagnosing to your doctor.

I do so myself. I've learned my lesson. I hope I've been able to impart it to you.

INDEX

293